Plant-Based High-Protein Cookbook

Nutrition Guide with 90+ Delicious Recipes

By Jules Neumann
Version 1.0
Published by *happyhealthygreen.life*
http://happyhealthygreen.life

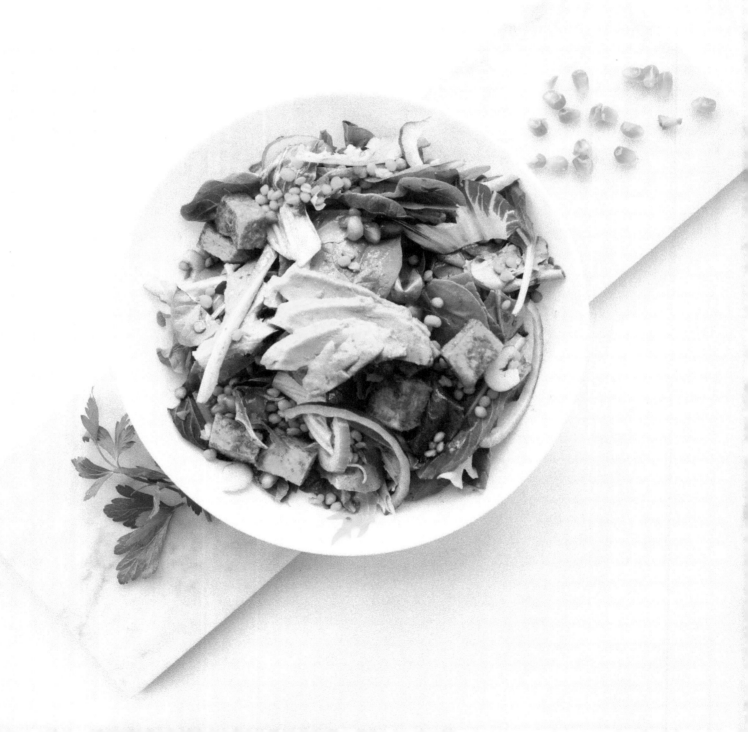

Introduction

It doesn't matter what your exact goals are, if you visit the gym, you want to see results. Weightlifters, athletes, and fitness enthusiasts usually have different objectives. That being true, if you're reading this book, you're most likely looking to improve your strength, build muscle, increase your endurance, or trim body fat. If that's the case, you'll need to eat right. Nutrition is essential to your workout success.

If you fail to supply your body with the nutrients and calories necessary for your fitness goals, you will never reach your full potential. That's why you want to manage your nutrition intake.

At this point of your journey, you probably need more than calories alone – you need a balance of nutrients to guarantee enough energy to cover your basic daily activities before exercise, plus the required nutrients for exercising and to guarantee muscle performance, recovery, and growth.

As intimidating as it sounds, working out while following a plant-based diet means having fewer food options than the average omnivore or even vegetarian. This is particularly true when it comes to the lean protein sources you need to build strength. Education is the best investment you can make as a vegan athlete, plant-based gym rat, or whatever label fits you.

Choosing the right foods and meals can be challenging, but this book will make it easy for you.

This book will also teach you everything you need to know about proper plant-based nutrition and its complimentary vegan supplementation for an active lifestyle. And most importantly, you'll get to make easy-to-store, high-protein recipes that are part of a simple, customizable meal plan for a full month, broken down in 30 separate days.

The information in this guide isn't limited to the plant-based athlete. It's highly beneficial to anyone who wants to understand basic (plant-based) nutrition principles and cook tasty, healthy whole food recipes.

Table of Contents

Disclaimer

The recipes provided in this report are for informational purposes only and are not intended to provide dietary advice. A medical practitioner should be consulted before making any changes in your diet. Additionally, recipe cooking times may require adjustment depending on age and quality of appliances. Readers are strongly urged to take all precautions to ensure ingredients are fully cooked in order to avoid the dangers of foodborne viruses. The recipes and suggestions provided in this book are solely the opinion of the author. The author and publisher do not take any responsibility for any consequences that may result due to following the instructions provided in this book.

Congratulations *on your responsible and health-conscious decision to read this book.*

We're excited you're connecting with us, and for the journey ahead of you.

We offer our readers the exclusive opportunity to subscribe to our newsletter. Dozens of readers are already enjoying our latest *(high-protein)* recipes, trendsetting articles, fitness-related tips and tricks right in their inbox.

Become a subscriber and we'll send you a PDF of *'The Vegan Cookbook'* as a welcome gift!

Subscribe here: **http://happyhealthygreen.life/newsletter**

(We hate spam and will never email you more than twice a week.)

Liking & following our Facebook page is also great to stay up-to-date and reach out. You can find our page here: **https://www.facebook.com/happyhealthygreen.life**

The Plant-Based Fitness & Vegan Athletes Facebook group is where you get connect with hundreds of other plant-based athletes, get inspired, share results and ask all your questions!

Join us here: **https://www.facebook.com/groups/PlantBasedAthletes**

See you inside!

The HappyHealthyGreen team!

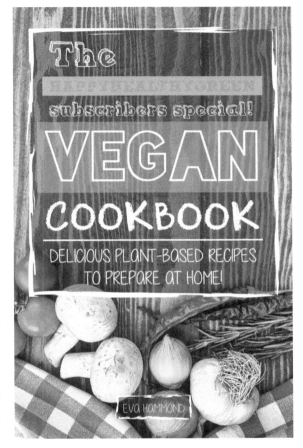

The Plant-Based Athlete

Athletes engage in strenuous and regular strength or endurance training with the goal of consistently improving their form and performance over time. Exercise should be followed by a period of recovery, aided by nutrition, to guarantee improvement.

Fueling your muscles on a plant-based diet doesn't have to be hard. A plant-powered athlete is able to get the same nutrients and arguably eats better than an omnivore sportsperson. Kendrick Farris (@kendrickjfarris), Patrik Baboumian (@patrikbaboumian), Jehina Malik (@ifbbjehinamalik1), and Nate Diaz (@natediaz209) are just a few of many famous, vegan athletes that have already proven this to the world.

The plant-based nutrients we'll discuss in the following pages are an essential part of recovery. If you don't take the necessary steps to rest and recover, your performance level will be hampered, and your progress will be compromised. Make sure to always work out recovered and with optimal energy. This way, your performance in the gym, at work, and at home will not suffer.

Energy and Performance

The body's preferred source of energy is glucose, which is generally derived from carbohydrates in your diet. Because carbs are easy to break down, they are often touted as a great energy source. Unfortunately, supplying your body with a healthy source of long-term energy is not as simple as binging on carbs. It's important to consume appropriate quantities of the right types of carbohydrates throughout the day.

SIMPLE CARBS VS. COMPLEX CARBS

There are two main categories of carbohydrates: simple and complex. Simple and complex carbohydrates are broken down by the body and then converted into glucose for energy. However, they break down at different rates due to their different chemical structures.

Simple carbs are much easier for the body to break down and convert than complex carbs. This means simple carbs are "absorbed" into your bloodstream at a faster rate. Complex carbs take longer to break down, so they provide a slower stream of glucose to the body. The delayed glucose uptake of complex carbs provides the body with an energy source that is more long-term and keeps energy levels stable throughout the day. This also helps you feel satiated for longer.

When blood sugar levels spike from the intake of simple carbs, a large amount of insulin is released into the bloodstream. Shortly after a large insulin spike, your blood sugar will often drop quite suddenly. When the blood sugar level is very low, you'll most likely experience a crash, or feelings of fatigue. Of course, this is far from ideal if you're on the way to the gym, so a diet rich in complex carbs is preferable.

To measure the effect an ingredient or food will have on blood-sugar levels, you can reference the glycemic index, which assigns ratings of 0 to 100 to carb-rich foods to indicate how much the food will affect a person's glucose level. A rating of 100 is equal to pure glucose. Low glycemic index foods include oatmeal, beans, and legumes, which have a GI score of 55 or less.

Fruit is often sweet but more complex than high GI-foods like potatoes or short grain rice. Most fruits are more complex because of their composition of both sugar and fiber. This combination causes the body to absorb the glucose in these foods differently. Fruits also contain a number of vitamins that improve body function and performance.

Note that fruits like dates are still very calorie-dense. These sweet fruits should be moderately enjoyed and especially during a calorie-cutting phase, a principle that will be explained later in this book, tracked alongside other meals and food.

Fruit juices, however, are usually packed with sugars, and the fibers present in the original fruit are generally removed from the juice. Juices can therefore cause major blood-sugar spikes. Even fruit juices with "no added sugars" often still contain large amounts of natural sugars. They can be just as sweet as soda and are not very satiating without the fruits' natural fiber.

Consuming carbohydrates at the right times of day will help your body maintain stable energy levels. An excellent way to guarantee the needed energy level for an upcoming workout is to consume a meal that is rich in complex carbs one or two hours before your training session. This will be the moment of the day that your body requires the energy the most.

Sticking to the dishes found in the included meal plan in this book, that is designed to be applicable for a wide audience, will guarantee that 40% of your total daily calorie intake comes from carbohydrates. This amount of carbs should keep your energy level high enough to sustain intense and demanding workouts and help you function throughout the day.

When fat loss, or trimming weight is the goal, restricting the intake of carbohydrates will make it easier to control your daily calorie intake. Many people also find that avoiding carbs first thing in the morning and consuming a protein- and fat-rich breakfast is a great way to start the day. This makes them feel satiated, which can help achieve a caloric deficit if desired.

Fats

Over the past three decades, the nutrition community and the media have asserted that fats are bad. The truth of the matter, however, is that the body needs fat. For one thing, fat is required to absorb certain fat-soluble vitamins like A, D, E, and K. We need fat for healthy skin and hair, as well as a protective insulator for vital organs.

There are two main types of fat, and both can be found in plant sources. Unsaturated fats are liquid at room temperature, and more often come from plant sources. Plant-based saturated fats are solid and found in avocados, nuts, olives, and oils. These are generally healthier than animal products

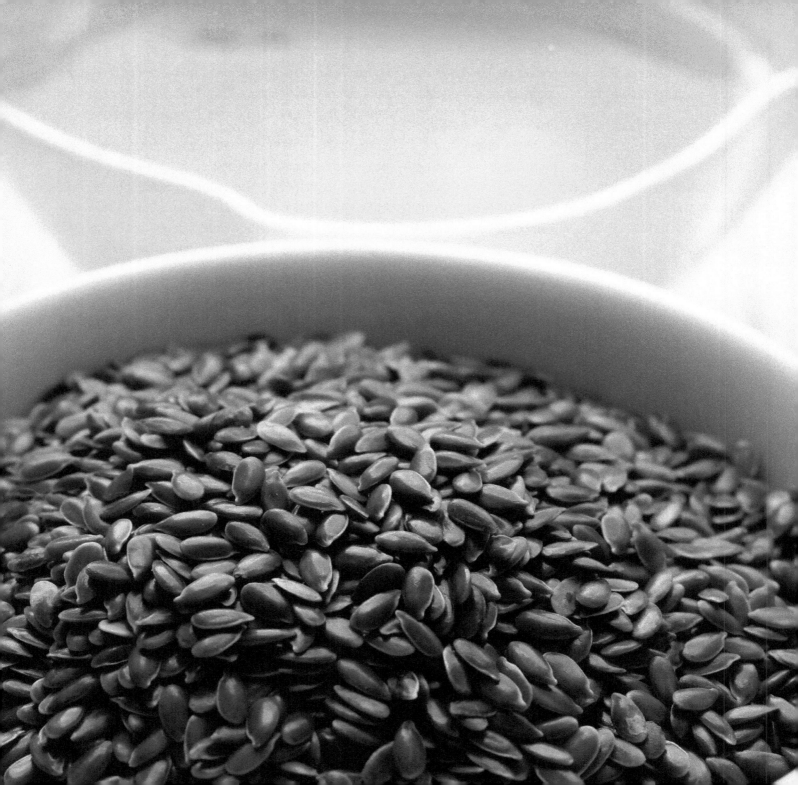

with saturated fats, which raise "bad cholesterol" (LDL) levels. LDL levels in the blood should always be less than 100 mg/dL. A plant-base whole food diet virtually guarantees very healthy LDL levels in the blood, since animal products are the only sources of dietary cholesterol.

HDL cholesterol helps remove other forms of cholesterol from your bloodstream and therefore is considered healthy in moderation. The suggested HDL levels in the blood range from 40 to 59 mg/dL. A plant-based diet rich in whole foods is HDL-friendly and foods include beans, legumes, whole grains, flaxseed, chia seeds, hemp seeds, nuts, avocados, fruits with a high fiber content, and soy-products.

In case you want to measure cholesterol levels in your blood, consult your doctor.

Trans fats are often produced by companies to increase the shelf life of their products. Trans fats are unsaturated fats that are turned into saturated fats by hydrogenizing the unsaturated fat. Needless to say, trans fats are bad and should be avoided at all costs. A diet rich in whole foods will make it easy to stay away from trans fats.

Omega 3-6-9

Fatty acids, essential fatty acids (EFAs), in particular -- alpha-linolenic (Omega-3) and linoleic acid (Omega-6) -- are intimately related to managing inflammation in the body. These fatty acids provide building blocks for your body to produce agents that increase and decrease inflammation in the body.

Your body is unable to produce Omega-3 and Omega-6 fatty acids, so it is critical that you consume ingredients that serve as a source for these fats. These essential fats help with numerous body processes like regulating blood pressure and brain development and functions.

Furthermore, fatty acids are vital for your body's functions, from your respiratory system to your circulatory system, which work together to circulate blood and oxygen throughout the body. Fatty acids are also essential to your brain and other vital organs. Ultimately, the body does produce the Omega-9 fatty acid, on its own.

The Omega-3 fatty acid is responsible for aiding brain function as well as preventing cardiovascular disease. It helps prevent asthma, certain cancers, arthritis, high cholesterol, blood pressure, and so on. The required dosage of Omega-3 can be satisfied by consuming sources such as chia seeds, walnuts, flaxseeds, hempseeds, and oil derived from these products. Alternatively, Omega-3 algae oil is available, which is vegan and high in the Omega-3 fatty acids DHA and EPA, which reduce inflammation and the risk of chronic diseases, like heart disease. DHA supports proper brain function and eye health.

Omega-6 can be found in various seeds, nuts, green veggies, and oils, such as olive oil. These fatty acids play a crucial role in brain function, and normal growth and development. Omega-6 fatty acids also help stimulate skin and hair growth, maintain bone health, regulate metabolism, and maintain the reproductive system.

The trick is to consume the right amount of fatty acids; aim to consume double the amount of Omega-6 fatty acid as the Omega-3. Doing so will prevent inflammation, as Omega-6 fatty acids are pro-inflammatory. A plant-based, whole foods diet virtually ensures a balanced intake of both fatty acids.

Lastly, the Omega-9 fatty acids are a non-essential fatty acid that the body can produce, but only when there are sufficient levels of Omega-3 and Omega-6 present, thus making it dependent on the consumption of the others. If your diet lacks the appropriate amounts of Omega-3 and Omega-6, then you can get additional Omega-9 from your diet or a supplement (since your body wouldn't be producing it in this case). Omega-9 fatty acids are naturally found in avocados, nuts, chia seed oil, and olive oil.

Protein & Recovery

Protein intake is crucial for repairing the muscle tissue that is worked during training sessions. Working the muscles creates micro-tears in the muscle tissue that need to heal before muscles can continue to grow. Proteins are necessary for the latter, as they are essentially building blocks for body tissues.

By eating the right amount of protein, your muscles will be able to recover and improve. Consuming enough calories and protein daily is crucial for hypertrophy, the increase of strength and size of muscles. Simply put, recovery and repair help your body adapt to an exercise.

The amount of daily protein intake required for repairing and gaining muscle after working out is 0.5-0.8 grams per pound of bodyweight, or 1,2-1,7 grams per kilogram. You can find the daily protein intake requirements for preserving muscle in the chapter 'Bulking and Cutting' on page 21.

Protein, depending on the source, is made up from different amino acid profiles. Amino acids compose many of the body's structures including nails, muscle, skin, and hair. 11 of the total 20 amino acids can be synthesized by the body and don't have to be obtained from food. The other 9, however, need to be present in your diet. All of these amino acids play a different role inside the body and even though only 9 are essential, a complete diet that includes all the 20 amino acids can enhance both your workout performance and recovery. Amino acids are also required for the production and availability of hormones in the body, which facilitate a number of vital functions in the body.

All 20 amino acids can be obtained from plant-based ingredients. Every ingredient that can supply the body with protein has a different amino acid profile. The nine essential amino acids are *leucine, lysine, tryptophan, isoleucine, histidine, valine, methionine, phenylalanine*, and *threonine*.

Beans and legumes contain high levels of *lysine* but are lacking in *methionine*. Examples include kidney beans, peanuts, peas, black beans, lentils, and garbanzo beans.

These sources can therefore be combined with grains such as rice that are high in *methionine*. Leafy greens like spinach, kale, broccoli, and romaine lettuce are high in *leucine*, *valine*, *phenylalanine*, and *lysine*.

A couple of exceptional plant foods are soy and quinoa. Both contain a great balance of amino acids. Soy even contains all nine essential amino acids, making it a complete protein source. And unlike many internet articles claim, soy is a perfectly responsible ingredient on a plant-based diet (soy allergy excluded). Daily requirements for amino acids are not extremely strict, since it's easy to get enough of every essential amino acid on a varied plant-based diet.

The following list is a breakdown of the nine essential amino acids, their functions, sources, and daily requirements:

✓ Lysine

Function: tissue growth, carnitine production

Daily requirements: 2000 - 3500 mg

Sources: beans, hemp, legumes (chickpeas and lentils), almonds, watercress, parsley, chia seeds, avocados, cashews, and spirulina

✓ Leucine (branched-chain amino acid or BCAA)

Functions: muscle growth and maintenance, blood sugar regulation

Daily requirements: 2000 - 3000 mg

Sources: peas, avocados, raisins, seaweed, pumpkin, whole grain rice, watercress, sesame seeds, turnip greens, kidney beans, figs, dates, blueberries, soy, apples, sunflower seeds, olives, and bananas

✓ Isoleucine

Functions: production of hemoglobin, energy production, muscle tissue repair

Daily requirements: 2000 - 3200 mg

Sources: brown rice, lentils, cabbage, rye, cashews, almonds, soy, sunflower seeds, sesame seeds, oats, beans, chia seeds, spinach, hemp seeds, pumpkin, pumpkin seeds, cranberries, blueberries, apples, quinoa, and kiwi fruit

✓ Methionine

Functions: cartilage formation

Daily requirements: 1050 - 1500 mg

Sources: whole grain rice, seaweed, beans, sunflower seeds, chia seeds, Brazil nuts, hemp seeds, oats, wheat, figs, onions, cacao, legumes, and raisins

✓ Phenylalanine (converted to tyrosine by the body)

Requirements: up to 8g (phenylalanine in supplement form should be avoided by pregnant women[1])

Daily requirements: hormone production precursor

Sources: quinoa, almonds, figs, leafy greens, spirulina, beans, rice, pumpkin, avocados, peanuts, most berries, raisins, and olives

---

1   https://www.ncbi.nlm.nih.gov/pubmed/818440

✓ **Threonine**

Functions: immunity, nervous system maintenance

Daily requirements: 1050-1500 mg

Sources: soybeans, sesame seeds, chia seeds, watercress, pumpkin, leafy greens, spirulina, hemp seeds, raisins, sunflower seeds, almonds, avocados, figs, quinoa, and wheat

✓ **Tryptophan**

Functions: mood regulation, sleep cycle regulation, circulation support, enzyme production, metabolism, and central nervous system regulation

Daily requirements: 280 – 350 mg

Sources: leafy greens, mushrooms, beans, figs, winter squash, oats, hemp seeds, chia seeds, seaweed, beans, beets, parsley, asparagus, all lettuces, avocados, celery, carrots, chickpeas, peppers, lentils, onions, oranges, bananas,

apples, spinach, soybeans, pumpkin, watercress, sweet potatoes, quinoa, and peas

✓ **Valine**

Functions: growth and repair of muscles

Daily requirements: 1600-2800 mg

Sources: soy, peanuts, chia seeds, whole grains, beans, legumes, broccoli, sesame seeds, spinach, cranberries, oranges, hemp seeds, avocados, apples, figs, blueberries, apricots, and sprouted grains

✓ **Histidine**

Functions: transportation of neurotransmitters

Daily requirements: 650 – 800 mg

Sources: wheat, beans, cantaloupe, hemp seeds, legumes, rice, rye, seaweed, chia seeds, potatoes, cauliflower, buckwheat, and corn

Protein Muscle Synthesis

Traditionally, protein is prescribed for consumption directly after a workout to maximize muscle recovery. Many people believe that muscle tissue continues to break down at a rapid rate after the completion of a workout and that this tissue should be replenished with protein within 45 minutes, so the muscles absorb the protein instantly and grow more as a result. This time period is often referred to as the "anabolic window".

However, this theory has been debunked. It's true that your muscles are still breaking down after a workout is completed, and that protein will help their recovery. But eating protein within 45 minutes is not necessary. Your body can utilize the protein from your last meal before the workout. A study conducted by the *Canadian Journal of Applied Physiology*[2] has shown that four hours after heavy resistance

2   https://www.ncbi.nlm.nih.gov/pubmed/8563679

training, the rate at which protein is synthesized in the muscles is elevated by 50%. After 24 hours, this rate increased to 109%. Not until 36 hours after the workout is the muscle protein synthetic rate returned to roughly its baseline.

In fact, as long as you are consuming enough protein throughout the day, there is no need to rush to your meal or shake straight after the completion of a training. As the research points out, the window in which protein is metabolized and then used for the growth of muscles is 4-36 hours. This time window can be even longer for new athletes, but usually shorter for experienced athletes or after a less stressful workout that has a lower impact on your muscles.

This window of elevated protein synthesis is essentially the time your muscles require to recover from a workout. For the best possible workout results, you should always aim to allow your muscles this period for proper recovery. You can start training a muscle or muscle group again after a 48-hour time window has passed. Beginners may require a longer recovery period and even experienced weightlifters, after a new training regimen or a change in technique, may also require an extended recovery period because they may stress the muscles in a new way.

Training your muscles before allowing them to recover completely can hamper your fitness results. The same is true for taking recovery breaks that are longer than necessary. Depending on your individual goals, you might want to train the same muscle (groups) multiple times a week. For the average person working out, training the muscles once or twice per week is fine, as long as you don't go more than a full week without a trip to the gym.

However, if you're serious about bodybuilding, you might want to work out every muscle every 48 hours. Note that it is always hard to measure the optimal recovery window precisely. There are a lot of variables involved that are not always under the control of the athlete, so a well-thought-out workout plan can help. For any input on your workout plan, join a growing number of plant-based athletes in our exclusive Facebook-group: https://www.facebook.com/groups/PlantBasedAthletes

For runners, or people that train for endurance, it is not necessarily to maximize the size or strength of the muscles. If you're serious about endurance, you want your workout plan to reflect that. Longer workouts deplete glycogen levels more than strength-oriented workouts, so consuming some foods with a higher GI (more simple carbohydrates), can help to restore your glycogen levels quickly after trainings.

CALCULATING AND TRACKING MACRONUTRIENTS

Macronutrients or "macros" is the name given to three groups of energy-dense nutrients that make up the most basic components of our diets: carbohydrates, fats, and proteins. In addition to acting as fuel, they facilitate many of our bodies' functions and are broken down by our digestive system for use in bodily structures. Each macronutrient provides us with the following number of calories:

- **1 g protein = 4 calories**
- **1 g carb = 4 calories**
- **1 g fat = 9 calories**

HOW DO YOU CALCULATE YOUR DAILY CALORIC INTAKE?

When preparing your meals, you will need to calculate two things: the macronutrients and the number of calories present in each meal. The recipes in this book take that responsibility off your shoulders; the included meal plan provides nutritional information for each day, with the correct balance of macronutrients and several options for different daily caloric intakes.

To benefit from the provided nutrition information, you need to know how much you need to eat in general each day. That's why we calculate daily caloric needs, also known as basal metabolic rate. This is essential for setting the bar for and keeping track of your daily macro intake. How to calculate your specific caloric needs is explained below.

This is the formula you need to use to calculate basal metabolic rate (BMR):

- **Men:** BMR = (9.99 x weight in kilograms) + (6.25 x height in centimeters) - 4.92 x age in years + 5.
- **Women:** BMR = (9.99 x weight in kilograms) + (6.25 x height in centimeters) - (4.92 x age in years) - 161.
- **Multiply the BMR number with the activity factor that fits your lifestyle.** With no exercise, your activity factor is 1.2. If you exercise one to three times a week, your activity factor is 1.375. If you engage in exercise three to five times per week, the activity factor is 1.55. For heavy exercise, six to seven times a week, the activity factor is 1.725. For athletes or those with heavy training sessions and/or a physically demanding job, your activity factor is 1.9. The number derived from this second calculation is the number of calories (kcal) required for maintaining a healthy weight.

Lowering your carb and fat intakes will allow you to burn fat more efficiently. For some athletes, a *carb to protein to fat* intake ratio of 50:25:25 is ideal. Once you have achieved your goals and wish to simply maintain your body weight, you want to focus on stabilizing your caloric intake with at least 15-20% of your calories coming from protein.

The following is a breakdown of how to achieve the 50:25:25 ratio on a 2000-calorie diet:

- 50% carbohydrates: 2000 x 50% = 1000 calories per day. To determine the amount needed, divide 1000 by 4 to get 250 grams of carbohydrates required daily.
- 25% protein: 2000 x 25% = 500 calories per day. Divide 500 calories by 4 to get 125 g of protein needed daily.
- 25% fat: 2000 x 25% = 500 calories per day. Divide 500 calories by 9 to get ~55.6 g of fat needed daily.

Tracking

Sticking to a meal plan and taking the time necessary to prep your meals will make the consumption of the proper number of daily macronutrients virtually effortless. By keeping a close eye on your carbohydrate, protein, and fat intake, your fitness goals will be within reach. Consciously tracking macros also makes it very easy to adjust your meal plan to address changing fitness goals and your body's needs.

Once you have a clear understanding of your daily calorie requirements, you can use this number to calculate the recommended number of daily macronutrients. As explained before, calories determine weight gain, loss, or maintenance. By consuming the correct ratios of macronutrients, you'll guarantee recovery and, combined with proper training, improve and optimize your muscular system and body composition.

Tracking macronutrients in this day and age is super simple thanks to apps like MyFitnessPal (https://www.myfitnesspal.com) and MacroTrak (iTunes) – (https://itunes.apple.com/us/app/macrotrak-macro-tracker/id1175925585?mt=8). If you don't have access to a smartphone or prefer a traditional or different method, tracking your intake by hand with a notepad or (digital) spreadsheet will work just fine.

Tracking effortlessly

The 30-day meal plan in this book further simplifies tracking calories. You only need to stick to the serving amounts of the recipes listed for each day, which eliminates the task of weighing portions. This meal plan covers a wide range of daily macronutrient targets so that you can plan for daily consumption of 1600, 1800, 2000, 2500 or 3000 calories, depending on your goals. Use this plan to your advantage!

The total number of macros you need to consume to reach your goals is based on your length, weight, and desired outcomes. You'll read more about this in the chapter "Bulking and Cutting". The daily calorie sums in the included meal plan, that is designed to appeal to a wide audience, are made up of roughly 30-35% protein, 35-40% of carbs, and 20-25% fats.

You can mix and match the daily plans to create a variety of week- or month-long plans easily without the need for recalculation. More info about using and customizing the 30-day meal plan in the chapter *'How to Use the Included Meal Plan'* on page 154. The only time you will need to record calories and macronutrients is when you eat something that is not part of your meal plan.

Whether you are trying to lose weight, maintain it, or gain muscle mass, the meal plan can be rearranged to align with your desired outcomes. You can read more about choosing the correct daily calories in the chapter *'Bulking and Cutting'* on page 21.

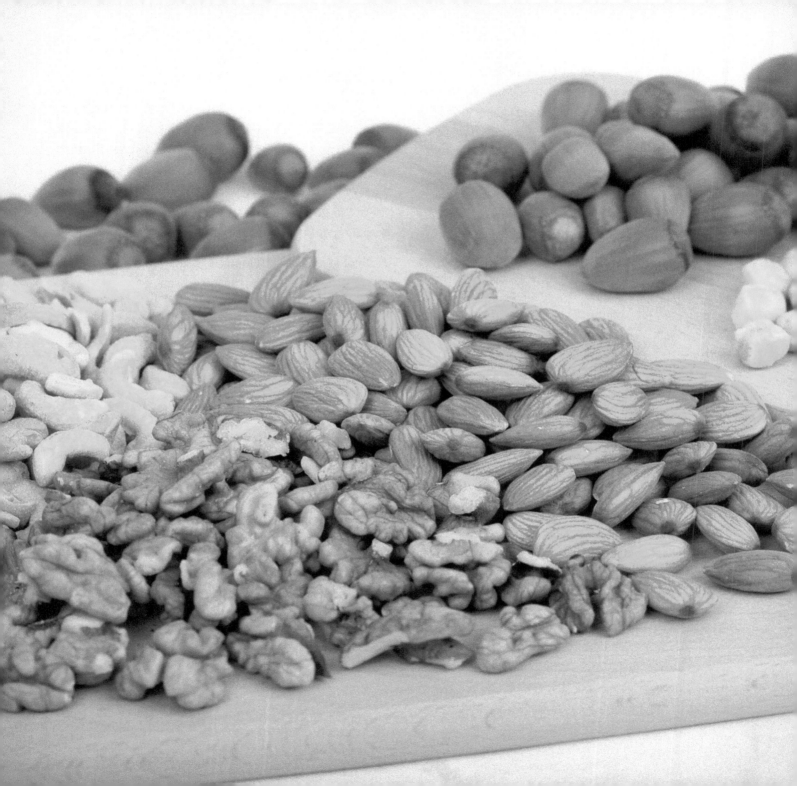

Plant-Based Protein Sources

Some great sources of plant-protein include tofu, tempeh, beans, lentils, and quinoa. The chart below shows some of the better plant-based (whole food) protein sources that are easy to store and their macronutrient breakdowns:

NAME	SERVING	PROTEIN	FAT	CARBS	FIBER
Hemp seeds, roasted	100 g	36.7 g	30 g	23.3 g	13.3 g
Hemp seeds, raw	100 g	33.3 g	46.6 g	6.7 g	3.3 g
Pumpkin seeds, roasted	100 g	32.1 g	46.4 g	14.3 g	10.7 g
Peanuts, roasted	100 g	26.7 g	50 g.	16.7 g	10 g
Peanuts, raw	100 g	26.7 g	50 g.	16.7 g	10 g
Split peas, dry	100 g	25.5 g	1 g	60.8 g	25.5 g
Pumpkin seeds, raw	100 g	25 g	46.4 g	17.85 g	3.6 g
Cranberry beans, dry	100 g	25 g	1 g	60.7 g	25 g
Seitan	100 g	24.6 g	3.5 g	7 g	1.75 g
Lentils, dry	100 g	24.4 g	0 g	60 g	15.55 g
White beans, dry	100 g	23.4 g	0.9 g	60.3 g	15.2 g
Sunflower seeds, raw	100 g	23.3 g	50 g	20 g	10 g
Kidney beans, dry	100 g	22.9 g	0 g	58.3 g	22.9 g
Lima beans, dry	100 g	21.6 g	0 g	62.7 g	21.6 g
Black beans, dry	100 g	21.6 g	1.4 g	62.4 g	15.2 g
Chickpeas, dry	100 g	21 g	13.15 g	60.5 g	18.4 g
Navy beans, dry	100 g	20.8 g	1 g	58.3 g	14.6 g
Pinto beans, dry	100 g	20.8 g	1 g	58.3 g	14.6 g
Sunflower seeds, roasted	100 g	20 g	50 g	20 g	10 g
Pistachio nuts, raw	100 g	20 g	46.7 g	30 g	10 g
Pistachio nuts, roasted	100 g	20 g	46.7 g	26.7 g	10 g
Tempeh	100 g	19 g	5.35 g	11.9 g	8.3 g
Pine nuts	100 g	15.4 g	65.4 g	11.5 g	3.8 g
Kamut	100 g	15 g	2.3 g	60.9 g	9.7 g
Oatmeal	100 g	14.3 g	7.1 g	67.85 g	10.7 g

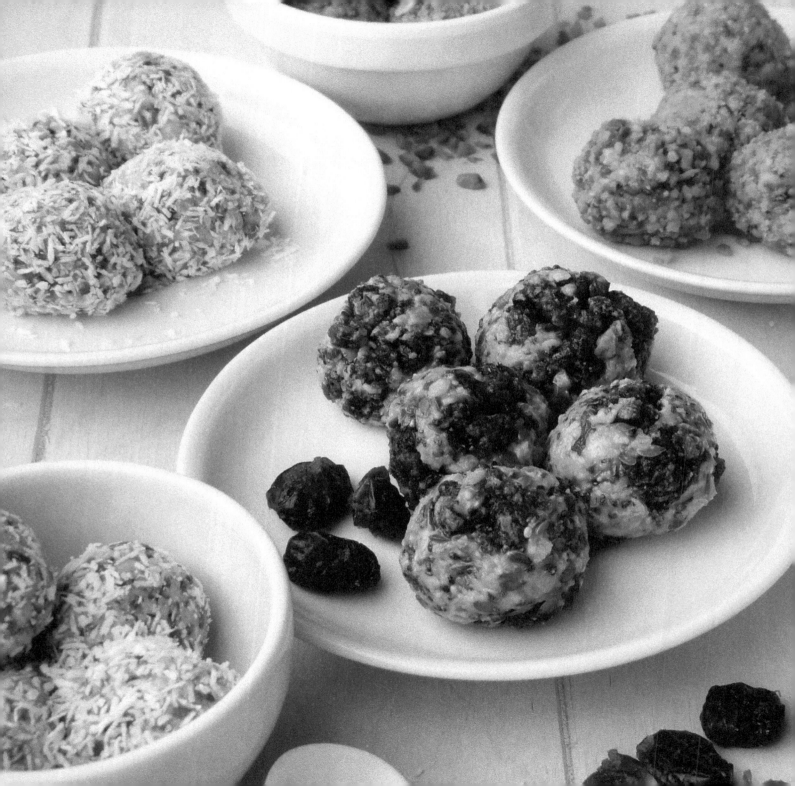

NAME	SERVING	PROTEIN	FAT	CARBS	FIBER
Yellow corn sweet, dry	100 g	14.3 g	3.6 g	67.85 g	21.4 g
Quinoa, dry	100 g	13.3 g	5.1 g	60 g	6.7 g
Buckwheat groats, dry	100 g	13 g	2.2 g	69.6 g	2.2 g
Edamame, raw	100 g	13 g	6.8 g	11.1 g	4.2 g
Soybean sprouts	100 g	12.9 g	7 g	9.4 g	2.35 g
Couscous, dry	100 g	12.8 g	0.6 g	77.4 g	5 g
Teff	100 g	12.2 g	3.65 g	70.7 g	12.2 g
Millet, raw	100 g	10.9 g	3.6 g	72.7 g	9.1 g
Edamame, cooked	100 g	10.9 g	5.2 g	9.9 g	5.2 g
White beans, cooked	100 g	9.7 g	0.4 g	25.1 g	6.3 g
Chickpeas, cooked	100 g	9.5 g	3 g	30 g	8.6 g
Tofu, firm	100 g	9.5 g	4.2 g	2.4 g	<1 g
Cranberry beans, cooked	100 g	9.3 g	0.5 g	24.5 g	10 g
Pinto beans, cooked	100 g	9 g	0.65 g	26.2 g	9 g
Lentils, cooked	100 g	9 g	0.4 g	20 g	7.9 g
Black beans, cooked	100 g	8.9 g	0.5 g	23.7 g	8.7 g
Kidney beans, cooked	100 g	8.7 g	0.5 g	22.8 g	6.4 g

Micronutrient Intake

Micronutrients (vitamins and minerals) play important roles in most of the body's functions. Vitamins fall into two categories: water-soluble (C and B complex) and fat-soluble (A, D, E & K) vitamins. Water-soluble vitamins are held in the body for up to three days and therefore need to be replaced through the diet regularly. Fat-soluble vitamins can be stored in the liver.

On a plant-based diet, particular attention needs to be paid to vitamin D, calcium, and vitamin B12. Vitamin B12, which plays a vital role in the procession of oxygen-carrying red blood cells, is predominantly found in animal products. Based on recommendations, an adult should consume 2.4mcg (µg) of vitamin B12 per day. On a vegan diet, it would be wise to supplement this and to be vigilant about consuming foods such as B12-fortified cereals. For more information, talk to your nutritionist or dietician about the best way to supplement.

Good plant sources of calcium include leafy greens such as collards and kale, as well as plant-based milk alternatives like soy, almonds, rice, and hemp milk. Vitamin D sources include portobello and shiitake mushrooms, as well as fortified plant-based milks. Though the best source of vitamin D is, of course, sunlight. If you live in a predominantly cloudy region of the world, it's a good idea to supplement.

DAILY MICRONUTRIENT REQUIREMENTS

Micronutrient	Recommended Dietary Allowance
Calcium	1200 mg
Phosphorus	700 mg
Magnesium	400 mg for men, 310 mg for women
Potassium	4700 mg
Sodium	1500 mg
Chloride	2300 mg
Iron	8 mg for men, 18 mg for women
Zinc	11 mg for men, 8 mg for women
Copper	900 mcg (µg)
Iodine	150 mcg (µg)
Manganese	2.3 mg for men, 1.8 mg for women
Vitamin A	900 µg for men, 700 µg for women
Vitamin D	15 mcg (µg)
Vitamin E	15 mg
Vitamin K	120 mcg (µg) for men, 90 mcg (µg) for women
Vitamin C	90 mg for men, 75 mg for women
Thiamine (B_1)	1.2 mg for men, 1.1 mg for women
Riboflavin (B_2)	1.3 mg for men, 1.1 mg for women
Niacin (B_3)	16 mg for men, 14 mg for women
Pantothenic acid (B_5)	1.3 mg
Pyridoxine (B_6)	1.3 mg
Biotin (B_7)	30 mcg (µg)
Folic acid (B_9)	400 mcg (µg)
Cobalamin/Vitamin B_{12}	2.4 mcg (µg)

Bulking and Cutting

Bulking and cutting are commonly used terms in the fitness and bodybuilding industry. The aim of bulking is to gain muscle mass, whereas cutting means to "cut" body fat while maintaining most of the hard-earned muscle mass. Bulking can be done "clean" or "dirty," while cutting follows stricter guidelines.

Whether you'll gain or lose weight will depends on your daily calorie intake. Everybody needs to consume a certain number of daily calories to support their daily activities and maintain their body weight. This number is known as the maintenance level or basal metabolic rate (BMR). It varies from person to person depending on genetic factors and levels of daily activity.

In order to bulk, you need to consume a larger number of calories than your maintenance level. This so-called calorie surplus will supply your body with the macronutrients it needs to be able to grow. On the contrary, for cutting you want to aim for a calorie deficit. This means consuming fewer calories than your maintenance level, which forces your body to rely partially on its stored energy.

Both bulking and cutting should be done at a constant, maintainable, healthy rate. There are alternative methods to cutting, like intermittent fasting, but those are not subject of this book.

Bulking

Bulking should always be done with as much "clean" food as possible, meaning mainly whole foods. This is fairly easy to implement on a plant-based diet. Consuming extreme amounts of calories and protein will only lead to increased stored fat. A constant, regulated surplus of calories will be less stressful for your body and manageable for the stomach.

When bulking, you want to aim for a constant increase in bodyweight. That increased caloric intake should be reflected in muscle and/or strength gains. Depending on your starting point, a gain of a half-pound to a pound per month is optimal. This range is often referend to as "lean bulking," which denotes a healthy and responsible way to

gain weight. Gaining a half-pound to one pound monthly can usually be achieved with a consistent calorie surplus of 15-20% above maintenance level.

An alternative way to bulk is "dirty bulking." This method simply comes to down to a large calorie surplus that will make you gain weight fast. Although everyone has individual motivations, this method is not very healthy or reliable. Therefore "dirty bulking" is not recommended here.

It takes time to repair and build muscle tissue. Although there are exceptions, if you are training naturally and gain more than a pound each month, you are likely eating too much and storing body fat, as well.

Cutting should be done according to similar principles. Losing weight too quickly is likely to lead to loss of precious muscle tissue and is usually unhealthy. Rapid weight loss happens with a calorie deficit that is too severe for the body to maintain its muscle mass. On average, a healthy rate of weight loss during a cutting phase should result in losing one to two pounds of body fat per week. This amount is always relative to the bodyweight of the individual.

In order to lose one pound of fat per week, you need to cut the equivalent number of that pound in calories from your diet. One pound of body fat is about 3500 calories, so you should aim to consume 3500 calories per week less than your maintenance level.

Bodyweight, genetic factors, and gender should always be taken into consideration while planning and working on a cut. In order to lose weight safely, you want to estimate a daily deficit number that fits both your goals and needs but doesn't affect your wellbeing.

Begin with your basal metabolic rate (BMR) of daily calories. For a week, weigh yourself every morning to accurately measure your total weight and then divide the total number by 7. Note that having access to a precise scale will give you more accurate results of what is happening with your body mass.

After this first week of weighing, you can start cutting down on calories. Start with a 5-10% deficit. For a female with a BMR of 1800 calories per day, this means lowering that number by 90-180 calories. The chart below indicates safe calorie numbers. Make sure to always calculate your BMR and work from there. Not one body is the same!

BMR	5% calorie deficit	10% calorie deficit	15% calorie deficit
1800	90	180	270
2000	100	200	300
2500	125	250	375
4000	200	400	600
5000	250	500	750

Increasing the consumption of protein during a cutting phase is a good idea for two reasons. First, the increased amount of protein keeps you satiated, so cravings will be less of a problem. Second, sufficient protein protects your muscle tissue and will result in a more catabolic cut, meaning better muscle preservation.

To minimize muscle loss during a cut, it's recommended to consume a slightly higher amount of protein (0.8-1 gram per pound, or 1,8-2,2 gram per kilogram of bodyweight.).

Nutrient requirements can virtually always be met with whole foods, but you can always get extra protein from protein shakes if needed. A shake is also the easiest meal to prep, but it is ultimately healthier to consume most of your nutrition in solid form.

Exercise

Cardio is many people's least favorite form of exercise, but it is a very effective way to promote fat loss. A serious cardio session combined with HIIT (high intensity interval training) can quickly and easily result in burning an additional 100-150 calories. Those burned calories can then be consumed on top of your BRM in the form of (mostly) protein to help preserve the hard-earned muscle mass.

Finally, make sure to track your results and weight constantly during the cutting phase. Make sure to drink a lot of water and pay extra attention to proper vitamin and fat intake. To keep your taste buds and stomach satisfied, choose one of the many delicious recipes from this book.

Plant-Based Supplements

First of all, supplements can aid recovery and progress but are never a magic pill. The right training, nutrition, and rest time are the real pillars for progressing physically. Supplements can give you an extra edge, but only if you're respecting these three pillars. Although a plant-based diet can cover all macro- and micronutrient requirements, it can be a challenge for serious athletes to prevent certain deficiencies. This is where vitamin and mineral supplements are a welcome addition to your diet.

Other types of supplements can help to improve your performance and recovery. As an athlete on a plant-based diet, you always want to confirm that supplements' manufacturing processes and ingredients are 100% vegan.

Amino Acids

As previously explained, most plant-based protein sources do contain a complete spectrum of amino acids. Still, it's very important to consume a wide variety of plant-based protein sources to ensure the right balance of amino acids in your diet[3].

Essential amino acid supplements can be very helpful. Branch-chain amino acids (BCAAs) are a great choice for vegan athletes. These supplements generally contain three of the essential amino acids: leucine, isoleucine, and valine. As we learned in the chapter 'Protein & Recovery' on page 10, these are required for proper protein synthesis.

BCAAs in supplement form are relatively cheap and cause no harmful side effects. The supplement is commonly produced as powder, which is often put in capsules to make consumption easier. A standard daily dosage for athletes is roughly 20 grams.

Another amino supplement that is beneficial before a workout is Citrulline malate. This supplement boosts the production of nitric oxide and enhances blood flow, nutrient uptake, and the transportation of oxygen. As a result, you'll experience a bigger "pump," meaning your muscles will swell more during a workout due to excessive blood flow. This blood carries all the nutrients necessary for the muscles to perform and will therefore enhance your capacity to exercise.

Creatine

Your body can produce small amounts of creatine by itself. Creatine[4] helps the muscle cells to produce more energy and improves performance for high-intensity exercises. Higher creatine concentrations have been shown to improve power output and delay muscular fatigue. Creatine can also increase the water content of muscles, speed up muscle growth, and may even battle Parkinson's and other neurological diseases.

Consuming five grams of creatine hydrate every day has been shown to increase the available energy inside muscles. When considering supplementing your diet with

---

3   https://www.ahajournals.org/doi/abs/10.1161/01.cir.0000018905.97677.1f
4   https://www.healthline.com/nutrition/10-benefits-of-creatine#section1

creatine, pre-load before the cycle starts since the body produces approximately only one gram per day. The creatine cycle consists of 3 phases:

1. Loading phase: 1 week; 5-20 grams of creatine each day.
2. Maintaining phase: 5-6 weeks; 3-10 grams of creatine each day.
3. Pause phase: 2-4 weeks.

In order to reap the benefits of creatine quickly, it's recommended to start with 20 grams of creatine per day[5] for about two days before the start of a workout cycle. On the third day – the first day of the workout cycle – the muscles will reach their maximum creatine storage capacity. From the third day on, a normal dosage of five grams of creatine per day is recommended.

If the 20 grams two-day pre-loading is not possible or desired, starting out with five grams per day also works. The maximum benefits will just take a few more days to occur.

Testosterone Boosters

A very interesting group of supplements is testosterone boosters that claim to increase natural testosterone levels. The androgen hormone is extremely important for muscle-building, body functions, and general wellness – the latter even more so for men.

Testosterone boosters that are targeted at vegans may claim that plant-based diets can lower testosterone levels. The opposite seems to be the case. A study published by the *British Journal of Cancer* points out that vegan men have 13% higher testosterone levels than men who eat meat on a regular basis[6]. To achieve this, it is extremely important to enjoy a varied and well-rounded plant-based diet that will not affect or hamper optimal testosterone levels.

Apart from anabolic steroids, many testosterone boosters do not provide a sufficient increase in free testosterone levels in the body to show any health-goal related benefits[7]. However, there are a few herbal and natural supplements that have shown positive results in boosting testosterone levels. These supplements may be especially interesting for people over the age of 40.

For example, D-aspartic acid [8]is a naturally occurring amino acid that is able to enhance the release of testosterone by an average of 42%. However, it has not shown a significant boost in active sportsmen and women. D-aspartic acid isn't useful as an athlete but could be if you're incapable of working out after a surgery or an accident and want to maintain higher testosterone levels.

Fenugreek

Fenugreek is an herb that boosts libido and raises testosterone levels in men. Fenugreek also increases insulin release, which can be helpful to increase blood flow and muscle mass

5   https://www.bodybuilding.com/content/do-i-need-to-load-with-creatine.html
6   https://www.ncbi.nlm.nih.gov/pmc/articles/PMC2374537/pdf/83-6691152a.pdf
7   https://www.healthline.com/nutrition/best-testosterone-booster-supplements#section1
8   https://www.healthline.com/nutrition/best-testosterone-booster-supplements#section1

after weight training. Fenugreek should be taken in dosages of 600 mg per day for it to produce the desired effects.

Ashwagandha

Another testosterone booster worth considering is ashwagandha. At the end of an eight-week study published in the *Journal of the International Society of Sports Nutrition*, 57 men saw their testosterone levels increase by an average of 18.7%. The herb is also able to help with muscle recovery, stress, anxiety, and cognitive function. 600-650 mg of ashwagandha is recommended daily to enjoy these benefits. To boost testosterone, dosages as high as 1,250 mg per day have been observed to yield positive results. Cycles with at least a week off every two to three months will prevent developing a tolerance.

Pomegranate

Pomegranate is also an interesting supplement. The fruit is loaded with antioxidants and works in several ways to help boost testosterone levels and performance. The Queen Margaret University of Edinburgh concluded that after two weeks of drinking a daily glass of pomegranate juice, 60 male and female volunteers aged between 21 and 64 saw an increase of salivary testosterone levels by 16-30%. The men had showed an average increase of 24%.[9]

Pomegranate also increases nitric oxide levels, which results in increased blood flow[10]. The fruit can be consumed whole or in juice or supplement form. The latter is the easiest (and a calorie-free) way to fit this fruit into your meal plan.

9   https://www.researchgate.net/publication/275716515_Pomegranate_juice_intake_enhances_salivary_testosterone_levels_and_improves_mood_and_well_being_in_healthy_men_and_women
10   https://www.anabolicmen.com/pomegranates-testosterone-and-erectile-quality

Cheat Days

From time to time, everybody starts craving certain foods. Snacks, fast food, and junk food are tempting to most people on occasion, though they sadly aren't very beneficial to an athlete's health (and performance).

While an occasional snack won't hurt, it is important to limit the consumption of foods that will not help you reach your goals. Following a meal plan that is in accordance with your individual needs is, with a meal prep approach, the only consistent path to positive results.

That said, completely banning foods that you like will usually lead to increased cravings for that food, so following a diet plan that is too strict can sometimes result in lost motivation and lower levels of adherence.

If the goal is to lose body fat (cut), cravings for these types of foods can be particularly hard to manage since they often contain a high amount of sugar and calories that are not beneficial to your objectives. Use these tips to manage your cravings better during a cutting phase:

- Increase your protein intake. High-protein foods are satiating and can stave off hunger for longer than other types of food.
- Increase your fiber intake. Insoluble fiber stays in its fibrous form, helps food pass through the digestive system, and makes you feel satiated faster without contributing any calories.
- Find alternatives for unhealthy foods. Substituting the snacks, fast food, and junk food with healthier alternatives will remove the feeling of being completely deprived. Allow yourself to try new, responsible snacks that are similar to, but healthier than the junk food you're craving. These often taste and feel better than any junk food you can think of and will curb your cravings.
- Drink more water. Thirst can sometimes be mistaken for hunger and drinking a glass of water can make cravings disappear. Wait 20 minutes after drinking to see if the craving is still there. Water will also make you feel satiated for longer and can reduce feelings of actual hunger.
- Stay busy. Boredom often results in cravings and keeping your mind active can help to reduce the temptation to eat as a distraction. Keep your mind focused on your goals and the much-desired outcomes from your diet.

Despite all the tips above, occasional feelings of the need to indulge a little may still occur. Planning cheat days or cheat meals will allow you to be flexible in a responsible way, while sticking to your diet.

As long as your caloric intake does not exceed your total daily allowance, and you consume the necessary number of proteins, your progress will not be affected by a cheat day every once in a while. Even during a cut, when you are generally consuming a lower number of calories than your maintenance level, a cheat day with some extra calories will simply bring you back up to maintenance level for a day. This may slow your progress slightly but won't completely derail it.

Monitoring your protein intake on a cheat day, however, is necessary to maintain hard-earned muscle mass. And again, the satiating properties of amino acids will reduce hunger and therefore somewhat limit the total number of calories you consume.

The best way to go about cheat days is to plan them properly. If you do go overboard and lose control, the best thing you can do for yourself is to accept your inaccuracy and get back on track with your meal plan immediately.

Keep working toward your goals. Again, as long as cheat days are occasional and don't become a regular part of your regimen, your progress won't be hampered.

Management and Fitness Goals

Time Management

The best diets and fitness plans are those that fit seamlessly into your daily life. Maintaining your health will always be a challenge if it takes too much time away from your normal activities. Common examples are work, family events, hobbies, and travel. Therefore, one of the most important parts of achieving your fitness goals is **planning** – to make the most productive use of the least time needed.

Athletes who want to increase performance, muscle mass or lower body fat percentage, can only get there through proper training, rest, and nutrition. The subject of this book is the latter, and this is arguably the most important component. Proper time management via planning meals will make the single biggest difference to your health if it is done right.

Planning Meals

A very simple way to save time and money and ensure results is to come up with an efficient meal planning routine. This process involves a (digital) calendar, diary, or app to remind you to shop and prepare your weekly meals. If prepping is done right, only one or two days of work per week are required to fuel a better body.

The consistent, daily intake of the correct number of macronutrients is absolutely vital to guarantee long-term physical progress. Most people consume three main meals every day and an additional two snacks to keep satiated

and energized throughout their waking hours. Eating every two to three hours helps to reduce hunger and keeps your energy level stable throughout the day. Different diet regimens like intermittent fasting are possible and can be beneficial, but these diet regimens are not the focus of this book. In case you are interested in plant-based fasting, you can send our Facebook page a message: (**https://www.facebook.com/happyhealthygreen.life**) or send us an email at **info@happyhealthygreen.life.**

The 30-day meal plan included in this book is exemplary but can be used exactly as it is. It plans out all your daily meals and snacks, and days can be repeated or re-ordered to last an unlimited number of weeks.

Although the 30-day meal plan can be followed as displayed, it's recommended that you customize it by combining various full-day plans to conform to your own preference and prepping regimen. This way, you'll only have to prepare 4-10 dishes for an entire week. How to do so will be covered completely in the chapter *'How to Use the Included Meal Plan'* on page 154.

Planning Workouts

Needless to say, workouts are very important. Too many people stumble into the gym with no real plan of action or direction. This most likely won't lead to any noticeable results. Sticking to a workout plan, whether strict or flexible, will point you in the right direction. Knowing what to do for how many sets and repetitions will make your workouts efficient and trackable. It will also help you save time and prevent worrying about being inefficient.

Most importantly, not having a plan means you won't have any means of tracking your progress, so it becomes very hard to see what is working for you and what may need to be changed. Progress is different for every individual and can come in many forms and degrees. For you, progress may be measured by mass gains, strength gains, or trimming body fat.

Usually you will be able to measure progress in more than one way: being able to lift heavier weights, complete a higher number of and better-controlled repetitions, take shorter rest periods, or perform more difficult exercises. Not unimportant is the aesthetic aspect of fitness that is inevitably related to measurable progress. The reflection in the mirror of a better, fitter, and stronger you can be very rewarding.

Make sure to track all these metrics over time. You can record all your workouts in a notebook, spreadsheet, or smartphone application. Once you have a workout plan and know what you need to do in order to reach your goals, you can head to the gym laser-focused. For any input on your workout plan (& nutrition), join a growing number of plant-based athletes in our exclusive Facebook-group (https://www.facebook.com/groups/PlantBasedAthletes)

Your custom, specific, measurable workout plan combined with the prepped meals will lead to the best, plant-powered version of you!

Soaking Methods and Cooking Staple Foods

Some plant-based whole foods come up time and again in various recipes and are good to have available in the pantry throughout the year. These ingredients are ideal as a base; they add texture, flavor, fiber, complex carbs, and protein to your meals. Amongst these staples are beans, grains, nuts, and seeds. These all contain phytic acid, a natural substance found in plant seeds that protects the seeds from insects or from sprouting too early. When people consume phytic acid, however, it impairs the absorption of important micronutrients like calcium, magnesium, copper, zinc, and iron.

In order to reduce the phytic acid in these foods, use soaking, sprouting, and/or cooking as a method to improve their nutritional value. Some foods are particularly high in phytates and are often consumed in large amounts on a plant-based whole-foods diet. Examples include almonds, sesame seeds, peanuts, soybeans, kidney beans, navy beans, and other types of legumes. **Therefore, reducing the phytic acids in ingredients with a large number of phytic acids is vital to avoid serious malnutrition and disrupted gut health.**

There are various ways to solve this problem. In general, beans and lentils are best soaked, sprouted, and/or cooked to get rid of phytic acids. Nuts need to be roasted, sprouted, or soaked. Buckwheat needs to be soaked and cooked. Grains like spelt or oats are best cooked for a longer period to get rid of the phytic acids. Sometimes fermenting is a preferred alternative to alter texture and get rid of most of the phytic acids. Soy products and chickpea tempeh are good examples of fermented products like this, but this book will not go into the details of that process.

Soaking

Soaking (dry) staples that are rich in phytic acids is absolutely necessary to guarantee proper nutrient absorption and a healthy gut. Most recipes in this book use raw beans, lentils, and nuts, which are very affordable to buy, effective to store and all easy to soak to effectively reduce their natural content of phytic acids. A popular and effective alternative to soaking is sprouting. Both methods are explained below.

1. Overnight soak

Leaving beans, lentils, and legumes in a pot filled with water overnight, meaning at least 8 hours, is the most effective way to soak. Use roughly 10 cups of water for every pound of dry beans or legumes (roughly 2 cups) and discard the excess water after the overnight soak. Recommended soaking times for different kinds are displayed in the chart below.

2. Hot soak

A quicker soaking method is to fill up a pot that is large enough to fit both the beans, lentils, or legumes and water. Use roughly 10 cups water for each pound (roughly 2 cups) of dry beans or legumes. Heat up the pot and bring the water to a boil. Once the water reaches a boiling point, immediately turn down the heat and allow the water to softly simmer for a few minutes. Continue to cover the pot, remove it from the heat, and allow the beans to sit for 1 to 4 hours. Discard the excess water after the hot soak.

Rinsing

After using the overnight or hot-soaking method, get rid of all the excess water that is left in the pot and rinse the beans or legumes once or twice with fresh, cool water. This will wash off any remaining indigestible sugars and phytic acids. After doing so, the soaked and rinsed beans or legumes are ready to be cooked.

Boiling

To boil beans and legumes, fill a pot that is large enough to accommodate the soaked beans or legumes with water. Make sure to cover the beans or legumes with an excess amount of water, which should be at least 1 inch. Partially cover the pot with a lid and put the pot over medium heat until the water is boiling. Aim for a soft boil and reduce the heat if necessary.

Note that both dry and canned Cannellini, white kidney, and red beans require to be boiled for at least a few minutes to get rid of the naturally present poison in these beans.

Cook the beans or legumes until soft. Cooking times vary for the kind of bean or legume that is being cooked, as displayed in the chart below. After cooking, make sure to drain the excess water. The cooked beans or legumes are now ready for consumption, to be incorporated in a recipe, or storage. Make sure that the beans or legumes are cooled before transferring them into a storage container and add some acidic ingredients like lemon juice, vinegar, or wine to prevent the cooked beans or legumes from becoming tender during storage.

SOAKING AND COOKING TIME PER BEAN OR LEGUME

*The recommended times in this chart are approximate.

Name (1 cup)	Soaking Time	Cooking Time	Yield (cooked, in cups)
Azuki Beans	4 hrs.	45-55 min.	3
Anasazi Beans	4-8 hrs.	60 min.	2 ¼
Black Beans	4 hrs.	60-90 min.	2 ¼
Black-eyed Peas	-	60 min.	2
Cannellini Beans	8-12 hrs.	60 min.	2
Fava Beans	8-12 hrs.	40-50 min.	1 ⅔
Chickpeas	6-8 hrs.	1-3 hrs.	2
Great Northern Beans	8-12 hrs.	1-½ hrs.	2 ⅔
Green Split Peas	-	45 min.	2
Yellow Split Peas	-	60-90 min.	2
Green Peas, whole	8-12 hrs.	1-2 hrs.	2

Name (1 cup)	Soaking Time	Cooking Time	Yield (cooked, in cups)
Kidney Beans	6-8 hrs.	60 min.	2 ¼
Lentils, brown	8-12 hrs.	45-60 min.	2 ¼
Lentils, green	8-12 hrs.	30-45 min.	2
Lentils, red or yellow	8-12 hrs.	20-30 min.	2 to 2 ½
Lima Beans (large)	8-12 hrs.	45-60 min.	2
Lima Beans (small)	8-12 hrs.	50-60 min.	3
Mung Beans	-	60 min.	2
Navy Beans	6-8 hrs.	45-60 min.	2 ⅔
Pink Beans	4-8 hrs.	50-60 min.	2 ¾
Pinto Beans	6-8 hrs.	1 ½	2 ⅔
Soybeans	8-12 hrs.	1-2 hrs.	3
Tepary Beans	8-12 hrs.	90 min.	3

A pressure cooker will reduce the amount of time required to cook beans and legumes. A 15-pound pressure cooker will cook beans or legumes about 6 times faster. In other words, what would normally take 1 hour, takes only 10 minutes. For a faster cooking time in a pot, adding Kombu seaweed during the overnight soak will halve the cooking time of beans.

If you're not sure whether something is ready to be consumed, you can test the beans or legumes. Stir well and take a few cooked beans from the pot, allow the beans to cool down and place them between your tongue and the roof of your mouth. Apply pressure with your tongue. If the beans "smoosh" easily, they are ready for consumption, to be used in a recipe, or stored after cooling down.

SPROUTING

An alternative way to prepare grains, nuts, seeds, beans, and legumes for consumption is sprouting. This means activating the germination in the seed. Sprouting takes longer than soaking and requires raw, unsprouted nuts, grains, seeds, or legumes. Germination increases the body's absorption of vitamins, beta-carotene, and some antioxidants. The process is also able to increase the availability of protein in various seeds and effectively reduces the anti-nutrient phytate by 37-81% in various types of grains and legumes.

Sprouting will also help to break down gluten, which helps the body with the digestion of gluten-rich staples. It makes the crude fiber content more available, which can otherwise not be absorbed by our digestive tracts.[11]

Start by rinsing the chosen seeds and cover these with cold water for 2-12 hours in order to soak. After soaking, discard the water and rinse the seeds, nuts, grains, or legumes. Ideally, the soaked seeds should then be exposed to air for

11   https://draxe.com/sprout

3-24 hours before being transferred into a sprouter. Sprouting will take various hours, depending on the kind. A deep plate covered by a lid or towel also works if you don't have a sprouter. Make sure to rinse the seeds every 8 to 12 hours during the recommended sprouting time and add about 2 tablespoons of water to the sprouter or deep plate after.

When the beans, grains, or legumes have sprouted a root, they are ready to be cooked. Alternatively, the sprouts can be kept in the fridge for up to 7 days. Doing so requires the sprouts to be rinsed every day in order to avoid mold or harmful bacteria growing.

A list of approximate sprouting times for some popular nut, seeds, beans, legumes, and grains:

Nuts and seeds:

- Almonds: 2-3 days
- Pumpkin seeds: 1-2 days
- Radish seeds: 3-4 days
- Alfalfa seeds: 3-5 days
- Pumpkin seeds: 1-2 days
- Sesame seeds: 1-2 days
- Sunflower seeds: 2-3 days

Beans and legumes:

- Chickpeas: 2-3 days
- Adzuki beans: 2-3 days
- Black beans: 3 days
- White beans: 2-3 days
- Mung beans: 2-4 days
- Kidney beans: 5-7 days

- Navy beans: 2-3 days
- Lentils: 2-3 days
- Peas: 2-3 days

Grains:

- Buckwheat: 2-3 days
- Amaranth grains: 1-3 days
- Kamut: 2-3 days
- Millet: 2-3 days
- Oats: 2-3 days
- Spelt & Rye: 2-3 days
- Barley: 2 days
- Quinoa: 1-3 days
- Rice: 3-5 days
- Wild rice: 3-5 days
- Black rice: 3-5 days
- Corn: 3-5 days
- Wheat berries: 3-4 days

SOAKING SMALL SEEDS

Just as with other, usually larger seeds, (nuts, grains, or legumes), soaking chia, hemp, and flaxseeds maximizes the availability of nutrients and aids their digestibility. These three small seeds are very common in plant-based diet.

To prepare chia seeds for consumption, place one part of seeds in a jar or glass and add six parts of water. Cover and shake the jar or glass or stir with a spoon for 2-3 minutes. To fully soak the seeds, allow the chia seeds to sit in the water for at least 1 hour. An extra stir or two during this time will aid the soaking process, as the seeds tend to stick together in lumps. An overnight soak in the refrigerator is the ideal way to get the gel-like pudding consistency of soaked chia seeds.

Tip: Use a mason jar to store the chia seeds in the fridge over longer periods of time. Since chia seeds do not go bad easily, it is possible to keep the seeds in the fridge for multiple days.

Hemp seeds are one of the most easily digested plant protein sources, and do not require soaking. The seeds can be consumed dry. If soaking is preferred, these nutritious seeds require a soaking time of 2-4 hours.

Flaxseeds don't absorb water the way chia seeds do but can be prepared in a similar way. These seeds in combination with water are an excellent vegan egg substitute and will function as a binder. To soak flaxseeds, put them in a jar or container and add double the amount of water as seeds. When working with ground flaxseeds, a 10-minute soak is enough for further use. Soak the flaxseeds for at least 2 hours when using whole seeds. After this time, the water will turn opaque from the soluble fiber and gums released by the flaxseeds. In case this liquid is not used in a recipe, it can be used to cook with and will add additional nutrients to a meal.

Sprouting small seeds

Sprouting smaller seeds like chia, hemp, and flaxseed is not the same as sprouting larger seeds. The smaller seeds have a mucilaginous coat, which will release soluble fibers when soaked in water. To activate the germination in these small seeds, rinse them well and put them into a shallow dish. Cover the dish with foil or a lid and place the dish in a sunlit area. Spray the seeds with fresh water twice a day to keep them moist. After 3 to 7 days, the seeds will start sprouting. Alternatively, use moist paper towels and refresh this at least once a day. Note that the wet seeds might stick to the paper towel when you try to replace it.

Rice

A very popular nutritious staple food is rice, which is available in many varieties. Each type of rice requires a slightly different preparation method. Brown rice, for example, requires more water and takes longer to cook than white rice. Rice can be prepared by using a rice cooker, pot, or steamer. The traditional pot method is explained in detail bellow.

Types of rice:

- Long-grain rice – fluffy, non-sticky grains (basmati, jasmine, and red cargo)
- Medium-grain rice – tender, moist and chewy (brown, rosematta)
- Short-grain rice – short and plump, sticks together (sticky, sushi, Valencia)

Rinse long- and medium-grain rice prior to cooking. This is necessary to get rid of excess starch. Short-grain rice does not require rinsing as the starch provides the desired stickiness for the dishes in which this type of grains are used.

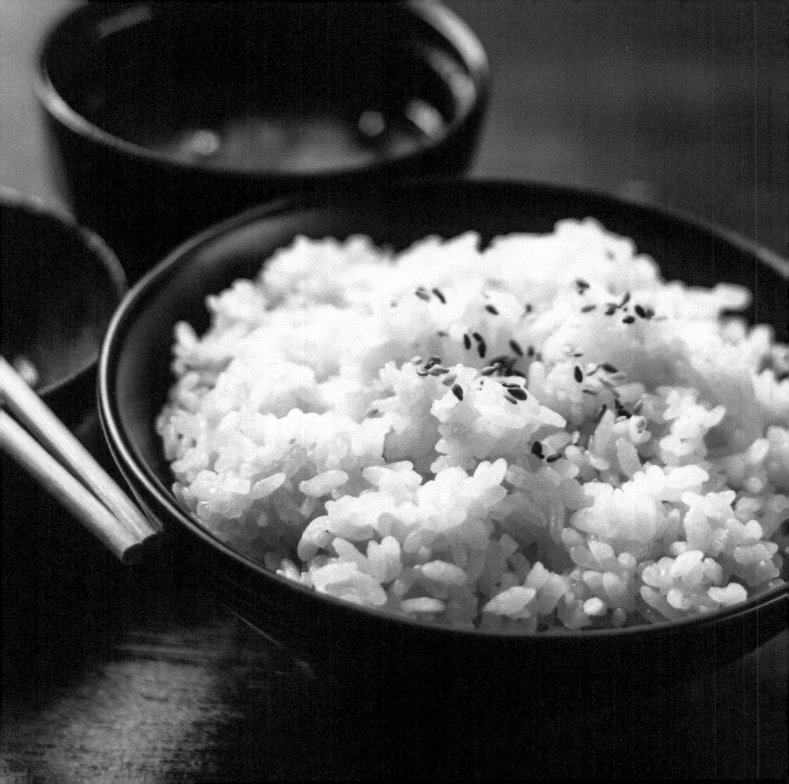

COOKING RICE IN A POT

LONG-GRAIN RICE:

1. Measure the rice by using a cup and level the top.
2. Rinse the rice in a strainer with cold water until the excess water is clear.
3. Optional: soak the rice for up to 30 minutes. Doing so will result in a shorter cooking time.
4. Pour the soaked rice into a pot and add two cups water for every cup of dry rice.
5. Optional: add a pinch of salt, oil, and other flavorings of choice.
6. Put the pot over medium heat and bring the water to a soft boil.
7. Put the lid on the pot and carefully shake it to distribute the rice evenly.
8. Cook the rice for 10 minutes with the lid on the pot and stir with a wooden spoon if necessary.
9. Once all water is absorbed, turn off the heat, remove the lid and cover the pot with a tea towel.
10. Set the rice aside to cool down before serving or using it in a recipe.

MEDIUM-GRAIN RICE:

1. Measure the rice by using a cup and level the top.
2. Rinse the rice in a strainer with cold water to get rid of grit, dust, and starch.
3. Add the rice into a pot and add two cups of water for every cup of (brown) rice.
4. Optional: add a little olive oil. This will improve the taste of brown rice.
5. Put the pot over medium heat, bring the water to a boil, lower the heat to medium-low, cover the pot and allow the rice to cook for about 45 minutes.
6. Check the rice. The majority of water should be absorbed, a little water left in the pot is fine. Drain excess water if necessary.
7. After cooking, allow the rice to rest with the lid on the pot for about 10 minutes.
8. Fluff the rice with a fork and set it aside for consumption or the recipe it will be incorporated in.

SHORT-GRAIN RICE:

1. Measure the rice by using a cup and level the top.
2. Wash the rice with a small amount of cold water to get rid of any surface dust.
3. Fill up a pot with the amount of water that is equal to the amount of rice used.
4. Soak the rice for at least 15 minutes and up to 3 hours.
5. Cover the pot with a lid, put it over medium heat and bring the water to a boil.
6. Once the water is boiling, turn the heat to medium-low.
7. Allow the water to simmer for about 15 minutes without removing the lid.
8. When all the water is absorbed turn off the heat and allow the rice to sit covered with the lid for 10 to 20 minutes.
9. Remove the lid and set the rice aside for consumption or another recipe.

Type of rice	Approximate amount of water required
White, long grain	1 ¾ - 2 cups per 1 cup rice
White, medium grain	1 ½ cups per 1 cup rice
White, short grain	1 ¼ cups per 1 cup rice
Brown, long grain	2 ¼ cups per 1 cup rice
Brown, medium grain	2 cups per 1 cup rice

For drier rice (Basmati or Jasmin), use slightly less water than displayed above.

QUINOA

Quinoa has a higher protein content than rice and is a common staple and tastes amazing in many plant-based recipes such as curry or salads. The superfood is easy to cook and just like rice, is available in several different varieties. Common examples are white, red, and black. White quinoa has a neutral flavor, while red and black have more distinct flavors and are often incorporated in salads. Preparation methods for the different types of quinoa are roughly the same.

METHOD FOR PREPARING QUINOA:

1. Measure the quinoa by using a cup and level the top.
2. Rinse the quinoa with cold water thoroughly and drain.
3. Transfer the rinsed quinoa to a pot and add two cups water for each cup of quinoa.
4. Put the pot over medium heat, cover it, and bring the water to a boil.
5. Occasionally stir the quinoa with a wooden spoon.
6. Turn heat down to medium-low and allow the quinoa to simmer covered for 15 minutes.
7. Take the pot off the heat and let the quinoa sit with the lid on top for 5 to 10 minutes.
8. Remove the lid and set the quinoa aside to cool down.

1. Cashew Cheese Spread

Serves: 1 cup of cheese / 5
servings | Prep Time: ~5 min |

Nutrition Information
(per serving)
- Calories: 151 kcal.
- Carbs: 8.8 g.
- Fat: 10.9 g.
- Protein: 4.6 g.
- Fiber: 1.0 g.
- Sugar: 1.7 g.

INGREDIENTS:
- **1 cup water**
- **1 cup raw cashews**
- **1 tsp. nutritional yeast**
- **½ tsp. salt**
- **Optional: 1 tsp. garlic powder**

Total number of ingredients: 5

METHOD:
1. Soak the cashews for 6 hours in water.
2. Drain and transfer the soaked cashews to a food processor.
3. Add 1 cup of water and all the other ingredients and blend.
4. For the best flavor, serve chilled.
5. Enjoy immediately, or store for later.

Tip: Substitute the raw cashews with oven roasted cashews to skip the soaking process and make roasted cashew cheese spread!

STORAGE INFORMATION:

Storage	Temperature	Expiration date	Preparation
Airtight container M	Fridge at 38 – 40°F or 3°C	4-5 days after preparation	
Airtight container M	Freezer at -1°F or -20°C	60 days after preparation	Thaw at room temperature

ESSENTIALS

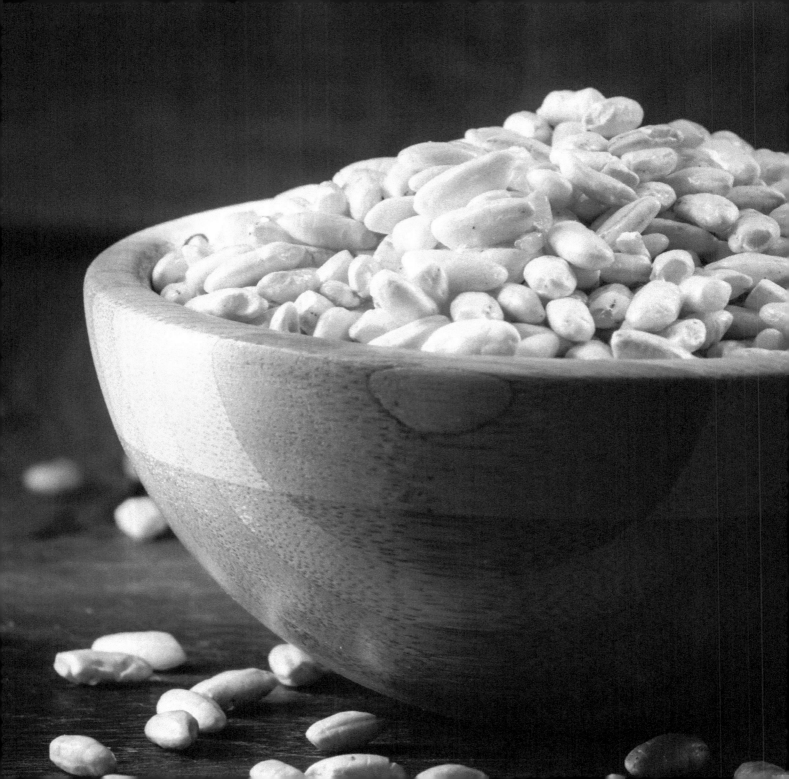

2. Puffed Brown Rice

Serves: 4 servings / 1 cup | Prep Time: ~15 min |

Nutrition Information
(per serving)
- Calories: 47 kcal.
- Carbs: 5.63 g.
- Fat: 2.48 g.
- Protein: 1.25 g.
- Fiber: 0.6 g.
- Sugar: 0 g.

INGREDIENTS:
- **½ cup brown rice (uncooked)**
- **4-8 cups of MCT oil**

Total number of ingredients: 2

METHOD:
1. Line a medium-sized bowl with paper towels. (This is for absorbing the excess oil after puffing the rice.)
2. Pour between 4-8 cups MCT oil in a medium-sized saucepan and heat over high heat; make sure that there is enough oil in the pan to cover an entire metal sieve.
3. Check if the oil is hot enough by throwing in a few grains. If these sizzle and puff up, the oil is hot enough.
4. Place the dry rice grains in the sieve and carefully lower it into the oil until it is fully covered. Shake gently to make sure everything puffs up. It will puff quickly so make sure to watch the process carefully; avoid burning the rice.
5. Remove the sieve with puffed rice and transfer the puffed grains into the bowl.
6. Let it cool down and discard the excess oil.
7. Use the puffed rice with a desired recipe and enjoy immediately, or store.

STORAGE INFORMATION:

Storage	Temperature	Expiration date	Preparation
Airtight container S	Fridge at 38 – 40°F or 3°C	4-5 days after preparation	
Airtight container S	Freezer at -1°F or -20°C	60 days after preparation	Thaw at room temperature

3. Sweet Cashew Cheese Spread

Nutrition Information
(per serving)
- Calories: 153 kcal.
- Carbs: 7.8 g.
- Fat: 11.4 g.
- Protein: 4.8 g.
- Fiber: 1.0 g.
- Sugar: 1.7 g.

INGREDIENTS:
- **5 drops stevia**
- **2 cups raw cashews**
- **Optional: ½ cup water**

Total number of ingredients: 3

METHOD:
1. Soak cashews for 6 hours in water.
2. Drain excess water and transfer the cashews to a food processor.
3. Add the stevia and, depending on the desired thickness, the optional water.
4. Blend until smooth.
5. For the best flavor, serve chilled.
6. Enjoy, use for another recipe, or store.

STORAGE INFORMATION:

Storage	Temperature	Expiration date	Preparation
Airtight container S	Fridge at 38 – 40°F or 3°C	4-5 days after preparation	
Airtight container S	Freezer at -1°F or -20°C	60 days after preparation	Thaw at room temperature

4. Peanut Butter

Nutrition Information
(per serving)
- Calories: 153 kcal.
- Carbs: 7.8 g.
- Fat: 11.4 g.
- Protein: 4.8 g.
- Fiber: 1.0 g.
- Sugar: 1.7 g.

INGREDIENTS:
- **2 cups raw peanuts (unsalted)**
- **½ tsp. sea salt**

Total number of ingredients: 2

METHOD:
1. Preheat the oven to 375°F / 190°C.
2. Roast the peanuts for about 10 minutes.
3. Transfer them to a food processor and process for about 1 minute.
4. Scrape down the sides of the food processor, add the sea salt, and blend again for 1 minute; continue until the desired consistency is reached.
5. For the best flavor, chill the mix before serving.

STORAGE INFORMATION:

Storage	Temperature	Expiration date	Preparation
Airtight container S/M/L	Fridge at 38 – 40°F or 3°C	5 days after preparation	
Airtight container S/M/L	Freezer at -1°F or -20°C	60 days after preparation	Thaw at room temperature

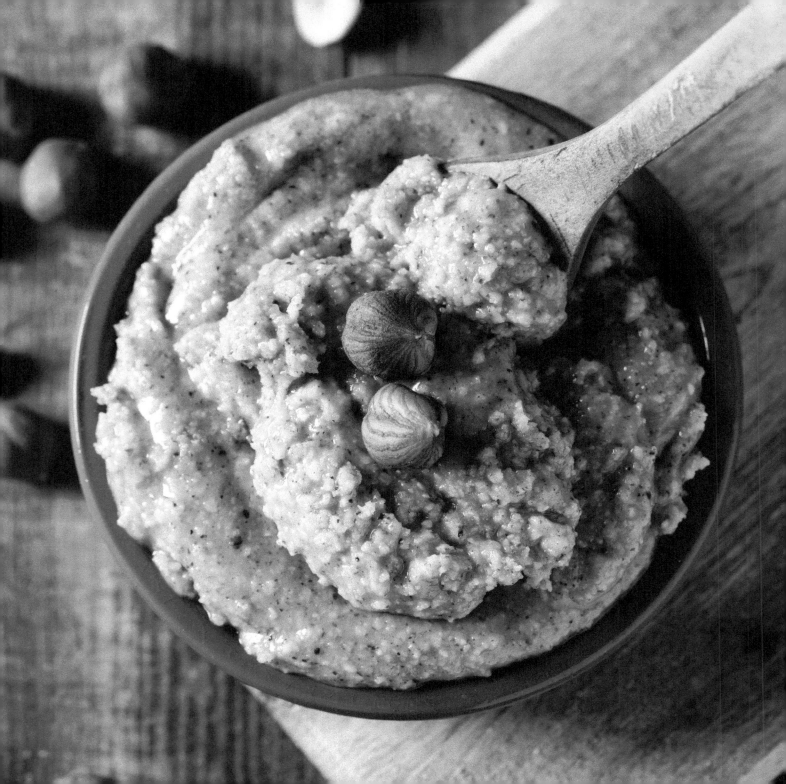

5. Chocolate Hazelnut Spread

Serves: 8 | Prep Time: ~20 min |

Nutrition Information
(per serving)
- Calories: 239 kcal.
- Carbs: 7.1 g.
- Fat: 20.6 g.
- Protein: 6.4 g.
- Fiber: 5.3 g.
- Sugar: 2.6 g.

INGREDIENTS:
- **2 cups raw hazelnuts (can be replaced with cashews)**
- **¼ cup coconut cream**
- **1-2 tbsp. cocoa powder**
- **1 tsp. stevia**
- **½ tsp. vanilla extract**
- **Optional: ¼ cup water**
- **Optional: ½ tsp. ground coffee beans**

Total number of ingredients: 7

METHOD:
1. Preheat the oven to 300°F / 150°C.
2. Roast the hazelnuts (or cashews) on a baking sheet lined with parchment paper.
3. After about 12 minutes, take out the nuts and let them cool down.
4. Put all the ingredients, including the optional ground coffee beans if desired, in blender or food processor.
5. Blend until smooth and add the optional water for a smooth mixture.
6. Stop and scrape down the edges of the blender or food processor if necessary.
7. Store, or use with another recipe and enjoy!

STORAGE INFORMATION:

Storage	Temperature	Expiration date	Preparation
Airtight container M	Fridge at 38 – 40°F or 3°C	5 days after preparation	
Airtight container M	Freezer at -1°F or -20°C	60 days after preparation	Thaw at room temperature

6. Pie Crust

Serves: 1 pie crust | Prep Time: ~40 min |

Nutrition Information
(per serving)
- Calories: 1157 kcal.
- Carbs: 131 g.
- Fat: 59.6 g.
- Protein: 24.2 g.
- Fiber: 19.7 g.
- Sugar: 1.7 g.

INGREDIENTS:
- **1½ cup whole wheat flour**
- **Pinch of sugar**
- **Pinch of salt**
- **¼ cup coconut oil (melted)**
- **¼ cup almond milk**

Total number of ingredients: 5

METHOD:

1. If preparing a fully cooked pie crust (rather than storing for later), preheat oven to 355°F / 180°C.
2. Combine the flour, salt, and sugar in a large bowl and mix well.
3. Add coconut oil and mix with a spoon until the mixture becomes a crumbly dough.
4. Blend in almond milk and mix again until everything can be formed into a ball of dough.
5. Roll out the dough on a flat surface covered with a tea towel. Use some flour to prevent sticking. Roll the dough out to be a bit larger than a pie dish.
6. Use the towel to flip the dough into pie dish and press it down. Cut down excess edges to form a nice crust.
7. Store for later or bake the crust for about 18 minutes until lightly browned.

STORAGE INFORMATION:

Storage	Temperature	Expiration date	Preparation
Ziploc bag or wrapping foil	Fridge at 38 – 40°F or 3°C	2-3 days after preparation	
Ziploc bag or wrapping foil	Freezer at -1°F or -20°C	60 days after preparation	Thaw at room temperature

Tip: Use almond, spelt, or coconut flour as an alternative for the whole wheat flour.

7. Flax Egg

Serves: 1 | Prep Time: ~10 min |

Nutrition Information
(per serving)
- Calories: 37 kcal.
- Carbs: 2.1 g.
- Fat: 2.7 g.
- Protein: 1.1 g.
- Fiber: 1.9 g.
- Sugar: 0 g.

INGREDIENTS:
- **1 tbsp. ground flaxseed**
- **2-3 tbsp. lukewarm water**

Total number of ingredients: 2

METHOD:

1. Mix the ground flaxseed with water in a cup.
2. Let the mixture sit, covered, for 10 minutes.
3. Use the flax egg in a recipe, or store.

STORAGE INFORMATION:

Storage	Temperature	Expiration date	Preparation
Airtight container S	Fridge at 38 – 40°F or 3°C	3-4 days after preparation	
Airtight container S	Freezer at -1°F or -20°C	60 days after preparation	Thaw at room temperature

Note: You can use this mixture to replace a single egg in any recipe.

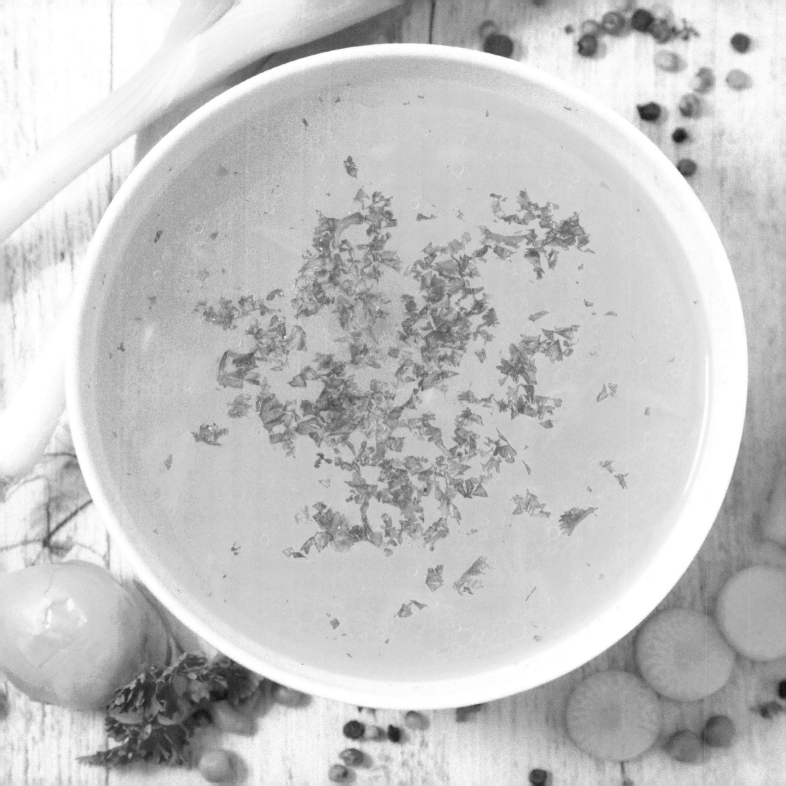

8. Vegetable Broth

Serves: 5 cups | Prep Time: ~90 min |

Nutrition Information
(per serving)
- Calories: 0 kcal.
- Carbs: 0 g.
- Fat: 0 g.
- Protein: 0 g.
- Fiber: 0 g.
- Sugar: 0 g.

INGREDIENTS:
- **10 cups water**
- **2 onions (chopped)**
- **3 medium garlic cloves (minced)**
- **4 carrots (chopped)**
- **3 leafless celery ribs (chopped)**
- **1 sweet potato (cubed)**
- **1 red bell pepper (sliced)**
- **1 cup fresh kale (or frozen, cut)**
- **½ cup fresh parsley**
- **½ cup olive oil**
- **1 tbsp. miso paste**
- **1 tbsp. thyme (dried)**
- **1 tbsp. rosemary (dried)**
- **Salt and black pepper to taste**
- **Optional: 2 tbsp. nutritional yeast**

Total number of ingredients: 16

METHOD:
1. Preheat oven to 400°F / 200°C.
2. Toss the onions, garlic, carrots, celery, sweet potato, bell pepper, kale, and parsley with the olive oil in an oven-proof roasting pan or baking tray.
3. Bake the veggies in the oven for about 20 minutes until browned and caramelized.
4. Put a large pot over medium heat and boil the water.
5. Add all ingredients from the roasting pan to the pot with boiling water.
6. Immediately bring the heat down to low and keep it at boiling point.
7. Stir every few minutes and add the miso paste, the optional nutritional yeast if desired, thyme, and rosemary.
8. Add salt, pepper, and any other desired spices to taste.
9. Cook until half of the water has evaporated.
10. Take the pot off the stove and let it cool.
11. Pour the mixture through a sieve and collect the broth in a second pot. Don't waste the veggies afterwards; they make for a nice side dish!
12. Use broth immediately, or store.

STORAGE INFORMATION:

Storage	Temperature	Expiration date	Preparation
Airtight container L	Fridge at 38 – 40°F or 3°C	5 days after preparation	Reheat in microwave or pot
Airtight container L	Freezer at -1°F or -20°C	60 days after preparation	Thaw at room temperature; Reheat in microwave or pot

Note: When freezing, divide the broth into smaller portions for convenient use later.

9. Vegan Half & Half Cream

Nutrition Information
(per serving)
- Calories: 106 kcal.
- Carbs: 2.4 g.
- Fat: 10.3 g.
- Protein: 1.0 g.
- Fiber: 0.7 g.
- Sugar: 0.8 g.

INGREDIENTS:
- **½ can full-fat coconut milk**
- **½ cup coconut cream**

Total number of ingredients: 2

METHOD:
1. Heat a small saucepan over low heat.
2. Pour the coconut milk in.
3. Cut up the coconut cream if necessary, and then add it to the coconut milk.
4. Keep stirring until the cream is dissolved.
5. Use warm or cold.
6. Enjoy immediately, refrigerate, or freeze.

STORAGE INFORMATION:

Storage	Temperature	Expiration date	Preparation
Airtight container S	Fridge at 38 – 40°F or 3°C	3 days after preparation	
Airtight container S	Freezer at -1°F or -20°C	60 days after preparation	Thaw at room temperature

10. Chili Garlic Paste

Serves: 12 | Prep Time: ~5 minutes |

Nutrition Information
(per serving)
- Calories: 116 kcal.
- Carbs: 5.9 g.
- Fat: 9.8 g.
- Protein: 1.2 g.
- Fiber: 2 g.
- Sugar: 0.8 g.

INGREDIENTS:
- ½ cup MCT oil
- 1 cup green chili flakes
- 2 medium garlic cloves (minced)
- 1 tsp. salt
- Optional: 2 tsp. sugar
- Optional: ¼ cup Szechuan peppercorns

Total number of ingredients: 6

METHOD:
1. Put all the ingredients into a blender or food processor and blend until smooth.
2. Store, or use right away with another recipe or as a topping.

STORAGE INFORMATION:

Storage	Temperature	Expiration date	Preparation
Airtight container S	Fridge at 38 – 40°F or 3°C	14 days after preparation	
Airtight container S	Freezer at -1°F or -20°C	60 days after preparation	Thaw at room temperature

11. No-Salt Cream Cheese

Nutrition Information
(per serving)
- Calories: 133 kcal.
- Carbs: 5.6 g.
- Fat: 10.9 g.
- Protein: 3 g.
- Fiber: 0.6 g.
- Sugar: 1.1 g.

INGREDIENTS:
- **2 cups raw cashews (unsalted)**
- **½ cup almond milk**
- **¼ cup olive oil**
- **½ tbsp. coconut vinegar**
- **1 tsp. nutritional yeast**

Total number of ingredients: 5

METHOD:
1. Fill a medium-sized pot with water and put it on the stove over medium heat.
2. Bring the water to a boil.
3. Place the cashews in the water and boil for up to 15 minutes.
4. Once cooked, strain the cashews and drain the excess water.
5. Place the cashews in a heat-safe blender container and blend until smooth.
6. Reuse the same pot and over low heat, bring the almond milk, olive oil, nutritional yeast, and vinegar to a simmer.
7. After 2 minutes, transfer the above mixture to a mixing bowl.
8. Slowly blend in the crushed cashews and stir the mixture into a smooth puree.
9. Mold into a block of cheese.
10. Enjoy right away, or store.

STORAGE INFORMATION:

Storage	Temperature	Expiration date	Preparation
Airtight container M or Ziploc bag	Fridge at 38 – 40°F or 3°C	3-4 days after preparation	
Airtight container M or Ziploc bag	Freezer at -1°F or -20°C	60 days after preparation	Thaw at room temperature

12. Cream Cheese

Nutrition Information
(per slice)

- Calories: 74 kcal.
- Carbs: 2.3 g.
- Fat: 6.8 g.
- Protein: 1.0 g.
- Fiber: 0.4 g.
- Sugar: 0 g.

INGREDIENTS:

- ½ tsp. sea salt
- 1 tsp. non-dairy probiotic powder
- 1 tsp. nutritional yeast
- 2 cups organic coconut cream (chilled)
- 1 tsp. garlic powder
- Optional: fresh herbs to taste

Total number of ingredients: 6

METHOD:

1. Whisk the salt, probiotic powder, yeast, and chilled coconut cream in a medium-sized bowl until smooth.
2. Wrap the mixture in a cheese cloth or coffee filter and place in a container or the previously used bowl; put it in the fridge for 24 hours.
3. After 24 hours, unwrap the cheese mixture, add the salt and garlic powder, and mix.
4. Cool the cheese in the fridge for another 6 hours.
5. Enjoy immediately, or store for later use.

STORAGE INFORMATION:

Storage	Temperature	Expiration date	Preparation
Airtight container M	Fridge at 38 – 40°F or 3°C	3 days after preparation	
Airtight container M	Freezer at -1°F or -20°C	60 days after preparation	Thaw at room temperature

13. Avocado Pesto

Serves: 2 cups / 8 servings | Prep
Time: ~5 minutes |

Nutrition Information
(per serving)
- Calories: 335 kcal.
- Carbs: 4.7 g.
- Fat: 36.1 g.
- Protein: 1.0 g.
- Fiber: 3.7 g.
- Sugar: 0.4 g.

INGREDIENTS:
- **2 ripe avocados (peeled and pitted)**
- **1 cup extra virgin olive oil**
- **1 cup fresh spinach**
- **¼ cup fresh basil**
- **2 garlic cloves**
- **1 tsp. black pepper**
- **1 tbsp. oregano (fresh or dried)**
- **1 tbsp. rosemary (fresh or dried)**
- **1 tbsp. parsley (fresh or dried)**

Total number of ingredients: 9

METHOD:
1. Combine all the ingredients in a blender or food processor.
2. Blend thoroughly until smooth.
3. Serve immediately and enjoy, or store for later.

STORAGE INFORMATION:

Storage	Temperature	Expiration date	Preparation
Airtight container M	Fridge at 38 – 40°F or 3°C	1-2 days after preparation	
Airtight container M	Freezer at -1°F or -20°C	60 days after preparation	Thaw at room temperature

14. Tortilla Wraps

Serves: 8 | Prep Time: ~20 minutes |

Nutrition Information
(per serving)
- Calories: 81 kcal.
- Carbs: 11 g.
- Fat: 4 g.
- Protein: 2 g.
- Fiber: 1.6 g.
- Sugar: 0 g.

INGREDIENTS:
- **2½ cups whole grain flour**
- **2 tbsp. olive oil**
- **½ cup water**
- **Pinch of salt**

Total number of ingredients: 4

METHOD:
1. Pour 2 cups of flour into a bowl.
2. Add the olive oil, water, and salt; mix well.
3. Add more water if the dough is too dry to mold and falls apart.
4. Make a big ball of dough and split into 8 equal parts.
5. Sprinkle a bit of flour on a flat surface for every ball.
6. Flatten the ball with your hands, and sprinkle flour on the ball of dough when it gets too sticky.
7. Use a dough roller to flatten the ball into a thin circle. Spin the dough often to prevent it from sticking to the surface.
8. Make sure that your tortilla wrap is thin and about the size of a medium plate.
9. Put a large pan over high heat and cook the tortilla for about 30 seconds.
10. Repeat the process for the remaining balls to make 8 delicious tortillas.

STORAGE INFORMATION:

Storage	Temperature	Expiration date	Preparation
Ziploc bag or wrapping foil	Fridge at 38 – 40°F or 3°C	3-4 days after preparation	
Ziploc bag or wrapping foil	Freezer at -1°F or -20°C	60 days after preparation	Thaw at room temperature

15. Hummus

Nutrition Information
(per serving)
- Calories: 97 kcal.
- Carbs: 13 g.
- Fat: 3 g.
- Protein: 4.6 g.
- Fiber: 3.5 g.
- Sugar: 2.5 g.

INGREDIENTS:

- **6 cups chickpeas (canned or cooked)**
- **3 tbsp. olive oil**
- **3 tbsp. tahini**
- **½ cup water**
- **3 tbsp. lemon juice (more to taste)**
- **½ tsp. cumin**
- **Salt and pepper to taste**

Total number of ingredients: 8

METHOD:

1. When using dry beans, prepare 2 cups of dry chickpeas according to the method on page 31.
2. Take a blender and add the chickpeas, tahini, olive oil, and the water.
3. Blend well until smooth.
4. Put all the remaining ingredients in the blender.
5. Blend all until smooth.
6. Transfer the hummus to a container and top it with some additional pepper and salt to taste.
7. Enjoy!

STORAGE INFORMATION:

Storage	Temperature	Expiration date	Preparation
Airtight container S/M/L	Fridge at 38 – 40°F or 3°C	4 days after preparation	
Airtight container S/M/L	Freezer at -1°F or -20°C	60 days after preparation	Thaw at room temperature

1. Cinnamon Apple Protein Smoothie

Serves: 1 | Prep Time: ~5 min |

Nutrition Information
(per serving)
- Calories: 373 kcal
- Carbs: 21.7 g.
- Fat: 10.3 g.
- Protein: 48.5 g.
- Fiber: 3.5 g.
- Sugar: 12.2 g.

INGREDIENTS:
- **1 green apple (peeled, cored, and chopped)**
- **1 cup coconut milk**
- **½ tsp. cinnamon**
- **2 scoops of vegan protein powder (vanilla flavor)**
- **Optional: 3 ice cubes**
- **Optional: 1-2 tsp. matcha powder**

Total number of ingredients: 8

METHOD:
1. Add all the required, and optional (if desired), ingredients to a blender.
2. Blend for 2 minutes.
3. Transfer the shake to a large cup or shaker.
4. Top with some additional cinnamon powder or sticks.
5. Serve and enjoy!

STORAGE INFORMATION:

Storage	Temperature	Expiration date	Preparation
Ziploc bag	Fridge at 38 – 40°F or 3°C	2-3 days after preparation	
Ziploc bag	Freezer at -1°F or -20°C	30 days after preparation	

This is a classic taste in a vegan smoothie—perfect if you love the apple / cinnamon combination.

BREAKFASTS

2. Tropical Protein Smoothie

Serves: 2 | Prep Time: ~5 min |

Nutrition Information
(per serving)
- Calories: 350 kcal
- Carbs: 44.4 g.
- Fat: 6.7 g.
- Protein: 27.9 g.
- Fiber: 5.8 g.
- Sugar: 30.5 g.

INGREDIENTS:
- 1 orange (peeled and parted)
- 1 cup mango chunks (frozen or fresh)
- 1 banana (frozen or fresh)
- ½ cup blueberries
- 2 scoops of vegan protein powder (chocolate or vanilla flavor)
- 1 tbsp. hemp seeds
- 6 ice cubes
- Optional: 1 tsp. guarana

Total number of ingredients: 8

METHOD:
1. Add all the required ingredients, and the optional guarana (if desired), to a blender.
2. Blend for 2 minutes.
3. Transfer the shake to a large cup or shaker.
4. Enjoy!

STORAGE INFORMATION:

Storage	Temperature	Expiration date	Preparation
Ziploc bag	Fridge at 38 – 40°F or 3°C	2-3 days after preparation	
Ziploc bag	Freezer at -1°F or -20°C	30 days after preparation	

Tropical goodness in a smoothie, packed with carbs, minerals, vitamins, and protein—this one is also perfect as a pre-workout.

3. Cranberry Protein Shake

Nutrition Information
(per serving)
- Calories: 325 kcal
- Carbs: 19.9 g.
- Fat: 16.8 g.
- Protein: 23.6 g.
- Fiber: 6.8 g.
- Sugar: 7.1 g.

INGREDIENTS:
- ¼ cup cranberries
- 2 scoops of vegan protein powder (chocolate or vanilla flavor)
- 1 banana (fresh or frozen)
- ¼ cup chia seeds
- ¼ cup hemp seeds
- 2 cups coconut milk
- 4 ice cubes

Total number of ingredients: 7

METHOD:
1. Soak the chia seeds according to the method on page 31.
2. Add all ingredients to a blender.
3. Blend for 2 minutes.
4. Transfer to a large cup or shaker and enjoy!

STORAGE INFORMATION:

Storage	Temperature	Expiration date	Preparation
Ziploc bag	Fridge at 38 – 40°F or 3°C	2-3 days after preparation	
Ziploc bag	Freezer at -1°F or -20°C	30 days after preparation	

Cranberry protein perfection... with healthy omega 3 fats and carbs to get that protein synthesis started, this smoothie is perfect as a post-workout.

4. Strawberry Orange Smoothie

Nutrition Information
(per serving)
- Calories: 287 kcal
- Carbs: 29.3 g.
- Fat: 7.5 g.
- Protein: 25.6 g.
- Fiber: 4.3 g.
- Sugar: 17.7 g.

INGREDIENTS:

- **2 cups coconut milk**
- **10 strawberries (fresh or frozen)**
- **1 orange (peeled and parted)**
- **1 banana (fresh or frozen)**
- **3 scoops of vegan protein powder (vanilla flavor)**
- **2 ice cubes**

Total number of ingredients: 6

METHOD:

1. Add all the required ingredients to a blender.
2. Blend for 2 minutes.
3. Transfer the shake to a large cup.
4. Stir and enjoy!

STORAGE INFORMATION:

Storage	Temperature	Expiration date	Preparation
Ziploc bag	Fridge at 38 – 40°F or 3°C	2-3 days after preparation	
Ziploc bag	Freezer at -1°F or -20°C	30 days after preparation	

Strawberries, orange, and protein—this smoothie is simple and great as a post-workout shake.

5. Powerhouse Protein Shake

Nutrition Information
(per serving)
- Calories: 257 kcal
- Carbs: 30 g.
- Fat: 3.5 g.
- Protein: 26.3 g.
- Fiber: 5.1 g.
- Sugar: 21.6 g.

INGREDIENTS:

- 2 green apples (peeled, cored, and chopped)
- 1 cup pineapple chunks (fresh or frozen)
- 1 cup kale (fresh, chopped)
- 1 cup spinach (drained and rinsed)
- 1 tsp. spirulina
- 1 cup coconut water (alternatively use 3-4 ice cubes)
- 2 scoops of vegan protein powder (unflavored)

Total number of ingredients: 7

METHOD:

1. Add all the required ingredients to a blender.
2. Blend for 2 minutes.
3. Transfer to a large cup or shaker.
4. Enjoy!

STORAGE INFORMATION:

Storage	Temperature	Expiration date	Preparation
Ziploc bag	Fridge at 38 – 40°F or 3°C	2-3 days after preparation	
Ziploc bag	Freezer at -1°F or -20°C	30 days after preparation	

This shake is full of antioxidant power and is ideal as a rest day / cleansing smoothie!

6. Avocado-Chia Protein Shake

Serves: 2 | Prep Time: ~10 min |

Nutrition Information
(per serving)
- Calories: 379 kcal
- Carbs: 16.6 g.
- Fat: 21.4 g.
- Protein: 30.1 g.
- Fiber: 9.8 g.
- Sugar: 2.8 g.

INGREDIENTS:

- **¼ cup chia seeds**
- **1 cup coconut milk**
- **½ avocado (pitted, peeled)**
- **1½ tbsp. peanut butter (page 43)**
- **2 scoops of vegan protein powder (chocolate flavor)**
- **1 cup water**
- **Optional: 3 ice cubes**
- **Optional: 1-2 tsp. cacao powder**

Total number of ingredients: 8

METHOD:

1. Soak the chia seeds according to the method on page 31. Drain any excess water.
2. Add all the required, and if desired, optional ingredients to a blender. When using ice cubes, the water can be left out.
3. Blend for 2 minutes.
4. Transfer the shake to a large cup or shaker.
5. Top with some additional cacao powder.
6. Serve and enjoy!

STORAGE INFORMATION:

Storage	Temperature	Expiration date	Preparation
Ziploc bag	Fridge at 38 – 40°F or 3°C	2-3 days after preparation	
Ziploc bag	Freezer at -1°F or -20°C	30 days after preparation	

A healthy, protein-rich "premium shake" full of nutrients, this shake is also low in carbohydrates.

7. Almond & Protein Shake

Serves: 2 | Prep Time: ~5 min |

Nutrition Information
(per serving)
- Calories: 340 kcal
- Carbs: 15.2 g.
- Fat: 17 g.
- Protein: 31.6 g.
- Fiber: 1.7 g.
- Sugar: 6.9 g.

INGREDIENTS:
- 1½ cup soymilk
- 3 tbsp. almonds
- 1 tsp. maple syrup
- 1 tbsp. coconut oil
- 2 scoops of vegan protein powder (chocolate or vanilla flavor)
- 2-4 ice cubes
- Optional: 1 tsp. cocoa powder

Total number of ingredients: 7

METHOD:
1. Add all the required ingredients, and if desired, the optional cocoa powder, to a blender.
2. Blend for 2 minutes.
3. Transfer the shake to a large cup or shaker.
4. Enjoy!

STORAGE INFORMATION:

Storage	Temperature	Expiration date	Preparation
Ziploc bag	Fridge at 38 – 40°F or 3°C	2-3 days after preparation	
Ziploc bag	Freezer at -1°F or -20°C	30 days after preparation	

8. Oatmeal Protein Mix

Nutrition Information
(per serving)
- Calories: 298 kcal
- Carbs: 24.7 g.
- Fat: 9 g.
- Protein: 29.3 g.
- Fiber: 3.9 g.
- Sugar: 2.2 g.

INGREDIENTS:
- **2 cups cooked oatmeal**
- **3 scoops of vegan protein powder (chocolate or vanilla flavor)**
- **½ tsp. cinnamon**
- **½ tsp. maple syrup**
- **¼ cup almonds**
- **1 cup oat milk (alternatively use almond milk)**
- **2 ice cubes**
- **Optional: 2 tbsp. peanut butter**

Total number of ingredients: 8

METHOD:
1. Add the required ingredients, including the optional peanut butter if desired, to a blender.
2. Blend for 2 minutes.
3. Transfer to a large cup or shaker and enjoy!

STORAGE INFORMATION:

Storage	Temperature	Expiration date	Preparation
Ziploc bag	Fridge at 38 – 40°F or 3°C	2-3 days after preparation	
Ziploc bag	Freezer at -1°F or -20°C	30 days after preparation	

This shake has it all: fats, protein, and carbs in a tasty drink... perfect for breakfast or a quick meal!

9. Almond Explosion

Serves: 4 | Prep Time: ~5 min |

Nutrition Information
(per serving)
- Calories: 355 kcal
- Carbs: 29.5 g.
- Fat: 15 g.
- Protein: 25.4 g.
- Fiber: 4.3 g.
- Sugar: 16.8 g.

INGREDIENTS:
- 1½ cup almond milk
  (unsweetened or homemade)
- 1 cup cooked oatmeal
- ½ cup raisins
- ½ cup almonds
- ½ cup water
- 3 tbsp. peanut butter
  (page 43)
- 3 scoops of vegan protein
  powder (vanilla flavor)
- Optional: ½ tsp. cinnamon
- Optional: 2 ice cubes

Total number of ingredients: 9

METHOD:
1. Add all the required ingredients, including the optional cinnamon if desired, to a blender.
2. Blend for 2 minutes.
3. Transfer the shake to a large cup.
4. Microwave the shake for a hot treat, or, add in the ice cubes and drink the shake with a straw.
5. Stir and enjoy!

STORAGE INFORMATION:

Storage	Temperature	Expiration date	Preparation
Ziploc bag	Fridge at 38 – 40°F or 3°C	2-3 days after preparation	
Ziploc bag	Freezer at -1°F or -20°C	30 days after preparation	

An explosion of almonds and protein... it's hard not to love this shake.

10. Banana Protein Punch

Nutrition Information
(per serving)
- Calories: 264 kcal
- Carbs: 23.3 g.
- Fat: 10 g.
- Protein: 20.2 g.
- Fiber: 4 g.
- Sugar:10.8 g.

INGREDIENTS:
- **2 bananas**
- **1 cup oat milk (alternatively use almond milk)**
- **½ cup almonds**
- **½ cup water (alternatively use 3-4 ice cubes)**
- **2 scoops of vegan protein powder (chocolate or vanilla flavor)**
- **Optional: 1 tbsp. maple syrup**

Total number of ingredients: 6

METHOD:

1. Add all the required ingredients, including the optional maple syrup if desired, to a blender.
2. Blend for 2 minutes.
3. Transfer to a large cup or shaker.
4. Enjoy!

STORAGE INFORMATION:

Storage	Temperature	Expiration date	Preparation
Ziploc bag	Fridge at 38 – 40°F or 3°C	2-3 days after preparation	
Ziploc bag	Freezer at -1°F or -20°C	30 days after preparation	

This shake guarantees a nice banana punch and is ideal after a training or workout session!

1. Lentil, Lemon & Mushroom Salad

Serves: 2 | Prep Time: ~10 min |

Nutrition Information
(per serving)
- Calories: 262 kcal
- Carbs: 28.1 g.
- Fat: 9.6 g.
- Protein: 15.8 g.
- Fiber: 14.8 g.
- Sugar: 9.3 g.

INGREDIENTS:
- ½ cup dry red lentils
- 2 cups vegetable broth (page 49)
- 3 cups mushrooms (thickly sliced)
- 1 cup sweet or purple onion (chopped)
- 4 tsp. extra virgin olive oil
- 2 tbsp. garlic powder (or 3 garlic cloves, minced)
- ¼ tsp. chili flakes
- 1 tbsp. lemon juice
- 2 tbsp. cilantro (chopped)
- ½ cup arugula
- Salt and pepper to taste

Total number of ingredients: 12

METHOD:
1. Sprout the lentils according the method on page 33. (Don't cook them).
2. Place the vegetable stock in a deep saucepan and bring it to a boil.
3. Add the lentils to the boiling broth, cover the pan, and cook for about 5 minutes over low heat until the lentils are a bit tender.
4. Remove the pan from heat and drain the excess water.
5. Put a frying pan over high heat and add 2 tablespoons of olive oil.
6. Add the onions, garlic, and chili flakes, and cook until the onions are almost translucent, around 5 to 10 minutes while stirring.
7. Add the mushrooms to the frying pan and mix in thoroughly. Continue cooking until the onions are completely translucent and the mushrooms have softened; remove the pan from the heat.
8. Mix the lentils, onions, mushrooms, and garlic in a large bowl.
9. Add the lemon juice and the remaining olive oil. Toss or stir to combine everything thoroughly.
10. Serve the mushroom/onion mixture over some arugula in bowl, adding salt and pepper to taste, or, store and enjoy later!

STORAGE INFORMATION:

Storage	Temperature	Expiration date	Preparation
Airtight container M/L	Fridge at 38 – 40°F or 3°C	3-4 days after preparation	
Airtight container M/L	Freezer at -1°F or -20°C	60 days after preparation	Thaw at room temperature; Reheat in pot or microwave

Note: Add a handful of spinach or other leafy greens for a heartier salad.

Tip: Use thickly sliced button or swiss brown mushrooms for the best results.

NUTRIENT-PACKED PROTEIN SALADS

2. Sweet Potato & Black Bean Protein Salad

Serves: 2 | Prep Time: ~15 min |

Nutrition Information
(per serving)
- Calories: 370 kcal
- Carbs: 48.8 g.
- Fat: 14.5 g.
- Protein: 11.4 g.
- Fiber: 10.6 g.
- Sugar: 8.6 g.

INGREDIENTS:
- **3 cups black beans (canned or cooked)**
- **4 cups of spinach**
- **1 medium sweet potato**
- **1 cup purple onion (chopped)**
- **2 tbsp. olive oil**
- **2 tbsp. lime juice**
- **1 tbsp. minced garlic**
- **½ tbsp. chili powder**
- **¼ tsp. cayenne**
- **¼ cup parsley**
- **Salt and pepper to taste**

Total number of ingredients: 12

METHOD:

1. When using dry beans, prepare 1 cup of dry black beans according to the method on page 31.
2. Preheat the oven to 400°F / 200°C.
3. Cut the sweet potato into ¼-inch cubes and put these in a medium-sized bowl. Add the onions, 1 tablespoon of olive oil, and salt to taste.
4. Toss the ingredients until the sweet potatoes and onions are completely coated.
5. Transfer the ingredients to a baking sheet lined with parchment paper and spread them out in a single layer.
6. Put the baking sheet in the oven and roast until the sweet potatoes are starting to turn brown and crispy, around 40 minutes.
7. Meanwhile, combine the remaining olive oil, lime juice, garlic, chili powder, and cayenne thoroughly in a large bowl, until no lumps remain.
8. Remove the sweet potatoes and onions from the oven and transfer them to the large bowl.
9. Add the cooked black beans, parsley, and a pinch of salt.
10. Toss everything until well combined.
11. Then mix in the spinach and serve in desired portions with additional salt and pepper.
12. Store or enjoy!

STORAGE INFORMATION:

Storage	Temperature	Expiration date	Preparation
Airtight container M/L	Fridge at 38 – 40°F or 3°C	3-4 days after preparation	Reheat in pot or microwave
Airtight container M/L	Freezer at -1°F or -20°C	60 days after preparation	Thaw at room temperature; Reheat in pot or microwave

Note: Add a variety of beans for more protein and flavor! Chickpeas, black eye, and navy beans are all great additions.

Tip: Use pre-cubed frozen sweet potatoes to reduce prep time.

3. Super Summer Salad

Serves: 2 | Prep Time: ~10 min |

Nutrition Information
(per serving)
- Calories: 371 kcal
- Carbs: 33.3 g.
- Fat: 20.8 g.
- Protein: 12.3 g.
- Fiber: 18.7 g.
- Sugar: 5.4 g.

INGREDIENTS:
Dressing:
- 1 tbsp. olive oil
- ¼ cup chopped basil (alternatively use parsley)
- 1 tsp. lemon juice
- Salt to taste
- 1 medium avocado (halved, diced) – use half for the salad
- ¼ cup water

Salad:
- ¾ cup chickpeas (canned or cooked)
- ¾ cup red kidney beans (canned or cooked)
- 4 cups raw kale (shredded)
- 2 cups brussel sprouts (shredded)
- 2 radishes (thinly sliced)
- 1 tbsp. walnuts (chopped)
- 1 tsp. flax seeds
- Salt and pepper to taste

Total number of ingredients: 14

METHOD:
1. When using dry beans, prepare ¼ cup of dry chickpeas and ¼ cup of dry kidney beans according to the method on page 31.
2. Soak the flax seeds according the method on page 31, and then drain excess water.
3. Prepare the dressing by adding the olive oil, basil, lemon juice, salt, and half of the avocado to a food processor or blender, and pulse on low speed.
4. Keep adding small amounts of water until the dressing is creamy and smooth.
5. Transfer the dressing to a small bowl and set it aside.
6. Combine the kale, brussel sprouts, cooked chickpeas, kidney beans, radishes, walnuts, and remaining avocado in a large bowl and mix thoroughly.
7. Store the mixture, or, serve with the dressing and flax seeds, and enjoy!

STORAGE INFORMATION:

Storage	Temperature	Expiration date	Preparation
Airtight container M/L	Fridge at 38 – 40°F or 3°C	4-5 days after preparation	Reheat in pot or microwave
Airtight container M/L	Freezer at -1°F or -20°C	60 days after preparation	Thaw at room temperature; Reheat in pot or microwave

Note: Add extra almonds, chopped parsley, or chia seeds for even more crunch and nutrients.

Tip: Add the water in 1 tablespoon increments to get the right consistency. Too much water will cause the dressing to be runny, and it won't stick to the other ingredients.

4. Roasted Almond Protein Salad

Serves: 4 | Prep Time: ~30 min |

Nutrition Information
(per serving)
- Calories: 206 kcal
- Carbs: 25 g.
- Fat: 7.4 g.
- Protein: 10 g.
- Fiber: 7.3 g.
- Sugar: 1.1 g.

INGREDIENTS:

- ½ cup dry quinoa
- 1½ cup navy beans (canned or cooked)
- 1½ cup chickpeas (canned or cooked)
- ½ cup raw whole almonds
- 1 tsp. extra virgin olive oil
- ½ tsp. salt
- ½ tsp. paprika
- ½ tsp. cayenne
- Dash of chili powder
- 4 cups spinach (fresh or frozen, alternatively use mixed greens)
- ¼ cup purple onion (chopped)

Total number of ingredients: 11

METHOD:

1. Cook the quinoa according to the method on page 38. Store in the fridge for now.
2. When using dry beans, prepare ¼ cup of dry navy beans and ¼ cup of dry chickpeas according to the method on page 31. Store in the fridge for now.
3. Toss the almonds, olive oil, salt, and spices in a large bowl, and stir until the ingredients are evenly coated.
4. Put a skillet over medium-high heat and transfer the almond mixture to the heated skillet.
5. Roast while stirring until the almonds are browned, around 5 minutes. You may hear the ingredients pop and crackle in the pan as they warm up. Stir frequently to prevent burning.
6. Turn off the heat and toss the cooked and chilled quinoa and beans, onions, and spinach or mixed greens in the skillet. Stir well before transferring the roasted almond salad to a bowl.
7. Enjoy the salad with a dressing of choice, or, store for later!

Note: Top with more almonds, walnuts, chickpeas, or kidney beans for even more plant proteins.

Tip: Use pre-roasted almonds to reduce prep time.

STORAGE INFORMATION:

Storage	Temperature	Expiration date	Preparation
Airtight container M/L	Fridge at 38 – 40°F or 3°C	3-4 days after preparation	Reheat in pot or microwave.
Airtight container M/L	Freezer at -1°F or -20°C	60 days after preparation	Thaw at room temperature; Reheat in pot or microwave

5. Lentil Radish Salad

Nutrition Information
(per serving)
- Calories: 247 kcal
- Carbs: 25.3 g.
- Fat: 10.7 g.
- Protein: 12.4 g.
- Fiber: 7.9 g.
- Sugar: 8.1 g.

INGREDIENTS:

Dressing:
- 1 tbsp. extra virgin olive oil
- 1 tbsp. lemon juice
- 1 tbsp. maple syrup (alternatively, use another sweetener)
- 1 tbsp. water
- ½ tbsp. sesame oil
- 1 tbsp. miso paste (yellow or white)
- ¼ tsp. salt
- Pepper to taste

Salad:
- 1½ cup chickpeas (canned or cooked)
- ¾ cup green or brown lentils (canned or cooked)
- 1 14-oz. pack of silken tofu
- 5 cups mixed greens (fresh or frozen)
- 2 radishes (thinly sliced)
- ½ cup cherry tomatoes (halved)
- Optional: ¼ cup roasted sesame seeds

Total number of ingredients: 15

METHOD:

1. When using dry chickpeas and lentils, prepare ½ cup of dry chickpeas and ¼ cup of dry lentils according to the method on page 31.
2. Put all the ingredients for the dressing in a blender or food processor. Mix on low until smooth, while adding water until it reaches the desired consistency.
3. Add salt, pepper (to taste), and optionally more water to the dressing; set aside.
4. Cut the tofu into bite-sized cubes.
5. Combine the mixed greens, tofu, lentils, chickpeas, radishes, and tomatoes in a large bowl.
6. Add the dressing and mix everything until it is coated evenly.
7. Top with the optional roasted sesame seeds, if desired.
8. Refrigerate before serving and enjoy, or, store for later!

STORAGE INFORMATION:

Storage	Temperature	Expiration date	Preparation
Airtight container M/L	Fridge at 38 – 40°F or 3°C	4-5 days after preparation	
Airtight container M/L	Freezer at -1°F or -20°C	60 days after preparation	Thaw at room temperature

Note: Extra sunflower seeds, roasted sesame seeds, or black-eyed beans taste great on this salad and add more nutrients!

Tip: If you don't have miso paste, you can replace it with the same amount of tahini.

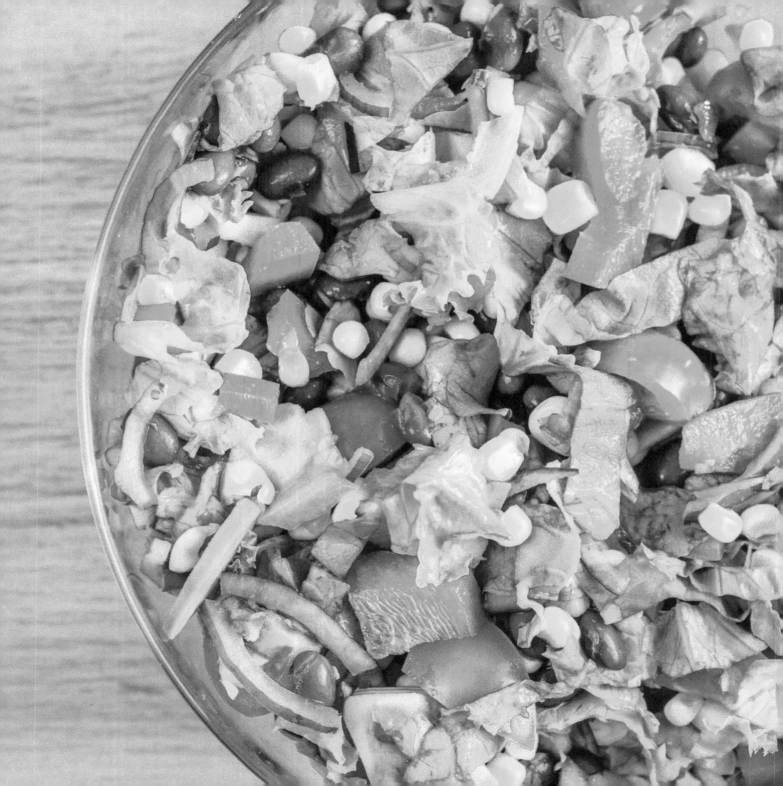

6. Southwest Style Salad

Nutrition Information
(per serving)
- Calories: 397 kcal
- Carbs: 51 g.
- Fat: 16.8 g.
- Protein: 11.2 g.
- Fiber: 13.2 g.
- Sugar: 7.6 g.

INGREDIENTS:

- 1½ cup black beans (canned or cooked)
- 1½ cup chickpeas (canned or cooked)
- ⅓ cup purple onion (diced)
- 1 red bell pepper (pitted, sliced)
- 4 cups mixed greens (fresh or frozen, chopped)
- 1 cup cherry tomatoes (halved or quartered)
- 1 medium avocado (peeled, pitted, and cubed)
- 1 cup sweet kernel corn (canned, drained)
- ½ tsp. chili powder
- ¼ tsp. cumin
- Salt and pepper to taste
- 2 tsp. olive oil
- 1 tbsp. vinegar

Total number of ingredients: 14

METHOD:

1. When using dry beans and chickpeas, prepare ½ cup of dry black beans and ½ cup of dry chickpeas according to the method on page 31.
2. Put all of the ingredients into a large bowl.
3. Toss the mix of veggies and spices until combined thoroughly.
4. Store, or serve chilled with some olive oil and vinegar on top!

STORAGE INFORMATION:

Storage	Temperature	Expiration date	Preparation
Airtight container M/L	Fridge at 38 – 40°F or 3°C	4-5 days after preparation	Reheat in pot or microwave
Airtight container M/L	Freezer at -1°F or -20°C	60 days after preparation	Thaw at room temperature

Note: Siracha or tabasco sauce makes a wonderful dressing for this smoky, southwest style salad.

Tip: Drain and dry the ingredients to prevent excess water/liquid. This will improve the taste and storage.

7. Shaved Brussel Sprout Salad

Serves: 4 | Prep Time: ~25 min |

Nutrition Information
(per serving)
- Calories: 396 kcal
- Carbs: 45.3 g.
- Fat: 18.7 g.
- Protein: 11.5 g.
- Fiber: 14.1 g.
- Sugar: 18.4 g.

INGREDIENTS:

Dressing:
- 1 tbsp. brown mustard
- 1 tbsp. maple syrup
- 2 tbsp. apple cider vinegar
- 2 tbsp. extra virgin olive oil
- ½ tbsp. garlic (minced)

Salad:
- 1½ cup red kidney beans (canned or cooked)
- ¾ cup chickpeas (canned or cooked)
- 2 cups brussel sprouts
- 1 cup purple onion
- 1 small sour apple
- ½ cup slivered almonds (crushed)
- ½ cup walnuts (crushed)
- ½ cup cranberries (dried)
- Salt and pepper to taste

Total number of ingredients: 15

METHOD:

1. When using dry beans and chickpeas, prepare ½ cup of dry kidney beans and ¼ cup of dry chickpeas according to the method on page 31.
2. Combine all dressing ingredients in a small bowl and stir well until combined.
3. Refrigerate the dressing for up to one hour before serving.
4. Use a grater, mandolin, or knife to thinly slice each brussel sprout. Repeat this with the apple and onion.
5. Take a large bowl to mix the chickpeas, beans, sprouts, apples, onions, cranberries, and nuts.
6. Drizzle the cold dressing over the salad to coat.
7. Serve with salt and pepper to taste, or, store for later!

STORAGE INFORMATION:

Storage	Temperature	Expiration date	Preparation
Airtight container M/L	Fridge at 38 – 40°F or 3°C	4-5 days after preparation	
Airtight container M/L	Freezer at -1°F or -20°C	60 days after preparation	Thaw at room temperature

Note: Toasted almonds and walnuts taste great with the sour apples, especially Granny Smith apples.

Tip: Shred the brussel sprouts very thinly for the best salad flavor.

8. Colorful Protein Power Salad

Nutrition Information
(per serving)
- Calories: 487 kcal.
- Carbs: 64.8 g.
- Fat: 15.5 g.
- Protein: 22.3 g.
- Fiber: 17.4 g.
- Sugar: 6 g.

INGREDIENTS:
- ½ cup dry quinoa
- 4 cups navy beans (canned or cooked)
- 1 green onion (chopped)
- 2 tsp. garlic (minced)
- 3 cups green or purple cabbage (chopped)
- 4 cups kale (fresh or frozen, chopped)
- 1 cup shredded carrot (chopped)
- 2 tbsp. extra virgin olive oil
- 1 tsp. lemon juice
- Salt and pepper to taste

Total number of ingredients: 11

METHOD:

1. Cook the quinoa according to the method on page 38.
2. When using dry beans, prepare 1⅓ cup of dry navy beans according to the method on page 31.
3. Heat up 1 tablespoon of the olive oil in a frying pan over medium heat.
4. Add the chopped green onion, garlic, and cabbage, and sauté for 2-3 minutes.
5. Add the kale, the remaining 1 tablespoon of olive oil, and salt. Lower the heat and cover until the greens have wilted, around 5 minutes. Remove the pan from the stove and set aside.
6. Take a large bowl and mix the remaining ingredients with the kale and cabbage mixture once it has cooled down. Add more salt and pepper to taste.
7. Mix until everything is distributed evenly.
8. Serve topped with a dressing, or, store for later!

Note: Add olive oil and apple cider vinegar for a simple dressing. It's a great compliment to all the flavors here!

Tip: Use purple cabbage if possible. The milder flavor tastes better raw compared to green cabbage.

STORAGE INFORMATION:

Storage	Temperature	Expiration date	Preparation
Airtight container M/L	Fridge at 38 – 40°F or 3°C	4-5 days after preparation	
Airtight container M/L	Freezer at -1°F or -20°C	60 days after preparation	Thaw at room temperature

9. Edamame & Ginger Citrus Salad

Nutrition Information
(per serving)
- Calories: 316 kcal
- Carbs: 38.9 g.
- Fat: 11.4 g.
- Protein: 14.4 g.
- Fiber: 15.4 g.
- Sugar: 10.4 g.

INGREDIENTS:

Dressing:
- ¼ cup orange juice
- 1 tbsp. lime juice
- ½ tbsp. maple syrup (alternatively, use a sweet substitute)
- ½ tsp. ginger, finely minced
- ½ tbsp. sesame oil

Salad:
- 1½ cup green lentils (canned or cooked)
- 2 cups carrots (shredded)
- 4 cups spinach (fresh or frozen, chopped)
- 1 cup edamame (shelled)
- 1 tablespoon roasted sesame seeds
- 2 tsp. mint (chopped)
- Salt and pepper to taste
- 1 small avocado (peeled, pitted, diced)

Total number of ingredients: 14

METHOD:

1. When using dry lentils, prepare ½ cup of dry lentils according to the method on page 31.
2. Combine the orange juice and lime juice, maple syrup, and ginger in a small bowl. Mix with a whisk while slowly adding the sesame oil.
3. Add the cooked lentils, carrots, kale, edamame, sesame seeds, and mint to a large bowl.
4. Add the dressing and stir well until all the ingredients are coated evenly.
5. Store or serve topped with avocado and an additional sprinkle of mint.

STORAGE INFORMATION:

Storage	Temperature	Expiration date	Preparation
Airtight container M/L	Fridge at 38 – 40°F or 3°C	4-5 days after preparation	
Airtight container M/L	Freezer at -1°F or -20°C	60 days after preparation	Thaw at room temperature.

Note: Substitute kale with any of your favorite mixed greens. Agave syrup can also be used instead of maple syrup.

Tip: Add the sesame seed oil slowly to prevent the dressing from separating.

10. Taco Tempeh Salad

Nutrition Information
(per serving)
- Calories: 441 kcal
- Carbs: 36.3 g.
- Fat: 23 g.
- Protein: 22.4 g.
- Fiber: 17.6 g.
- Sugar: 4.1 g.

INGREDIENTS:
- **3 cup black beans (canned or cooked)**
- **1 8-oz. package tempeh**
- **1 tbsp. lime or lemon juice**
- **2 tbsp. extra virgin olive oil**
- **1 tsp. maple syrup**
- **½ tsp. chili powder**
- **¼ tsp. cumin**
- **¼ tsp. paprika**
- **1 large bunch of kale (fresh or frozen, chopped)**
- **1 large avocado (peeled, pitted, diced)**
- **½ cup salsa (page 187)**
- **Salt and pepper to taste**

Total number of ingredients: 13

METHOD:
1. When using dry beans, prepare 1 cup of dry beans according to the method on page 31.
2. Cut the tempeh into ¼-inch cubes, place in a bowl, and then add the lime or lemon juice, 1 tablespoon of olive oil, maple syrup, chili powder, cumin, and paprika.
3. Stir well and let the tempeh marinate in the fridge for at least 1 hour, up to 12 hours.
4. Heat the remaining 1 tablespoon of olive oil in a frying pan over medium heat.
5. Add the marinated tempeh mixture and cook until brown and crispy on both sides, around 10 minutes.
6. Put the chopped kale in a bowl with the cooked beans and prepared tempeh.
7. Store, or serve the salad immediately, topped with salsa, avocado, and salt and pepper to taste.

STORAGE INFORMATION:

Storage	Temperature	Expiration date	Preparation
Airtight container M/L	Fridge at 38 – 40°F or 3°C	3-4 days after preparation	
Airtight container M/L	Freezer at -1°F or -20°C	60 days after preparation	Thaw at room temperature

Note: You can also serve this salad with tortilla strips and vegan cheese on top.

Tip: Marinate the tempeh longer for more flavor.

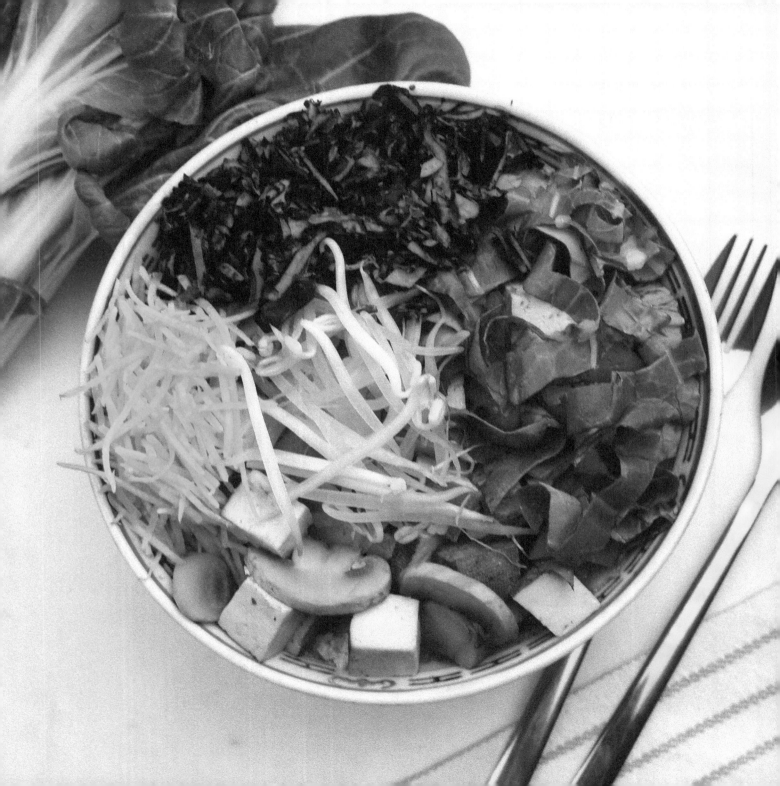

1. Mushroom Pho

Nutrition Information
(per serving)
- Calories: 383 kcal
- Carbs: 57.3 g.
- Fat: 9.1 g.
- Protein: 17.8 g.
- Fiber: 9.4 g.
- Sugar: 3 g.

INGREDIENTS:
- 1 14-oz. block firm tofu (drained)
- 6 cups vegetable broth (page 49)
- 3 green onions (thinly sliced)
- 1 tsp. or ½-inch minced ginger
- 1 tbsp. olive oil
- 3 cups mushrooms (sliced)
- 2 tbsp. hoisin sauce
- 1 tbsp. sesame oil
- 2 cups gluten-free rice noodles
- 1 cup raw bean sprouts
- 1 cup matchstick carrots
- 1 cup bok choy (chopped, optional)
- 1 cup cabbage (chopped, optional)
- Salt and pepper to taste

Total number of ingredients: 15

METHOD:

1. Cut the tofu into ¼-inch cubes and set it aside.
2. Take a deep saucepan and heat the vegetable broth, green onions, and ginger over medium high heat.
3. Boil for 1 minute before reducing the heat to low; then cover the saucepan with a lid and let it simmer for 20 minutes.
4. Take another frying pan and heat the olive oil in it over medium-high heat.
5. Add the sliced mushrooms to the frying pan and cook until they are tender, for about 5 minutes.
6. Add the tofu, hoisin sauce, and sesame oil to the mushrooms.
7. Heat until the sauce thickens (around 5 minutes) and remove the frying pan from the heat.
8. Prepare the gluten-free rice noodles according to the package instructions.
9. Top the rice noodles with a scoop of the tofu mushroom mixture, a generous amount of broth, and the bean sprouts.
10. Add the carrots, and optional cabbage and/or bok choy (if desired), right before serving.
11. Top with salt and pepper to taste and enjoy, or, store ingredients separately!

Note: For authentic pho flavors, add lime juice, cilantro, and basil as a garnish. For a spicier pho, add sliced jalapeños or sriracha!

Tip: Use low-sodium hoisin and broth to reduce salt intake. Store the noodles, tofu mushroom mixture, and broth separately.

STORAGE INFORMATION:

Storage	Temperature	Expiration date	Preparation
3-compartment airtight container M/L	Fridge at 38 – 40°F or 3°C	4-5 days after preparation	Reheat on stove or in microwave
3-compartment airtight container M/L	Freezer at -1°F or -20°C	60 days after preparation	Thaw at room temperature; Reheat in a pot or in the microwave

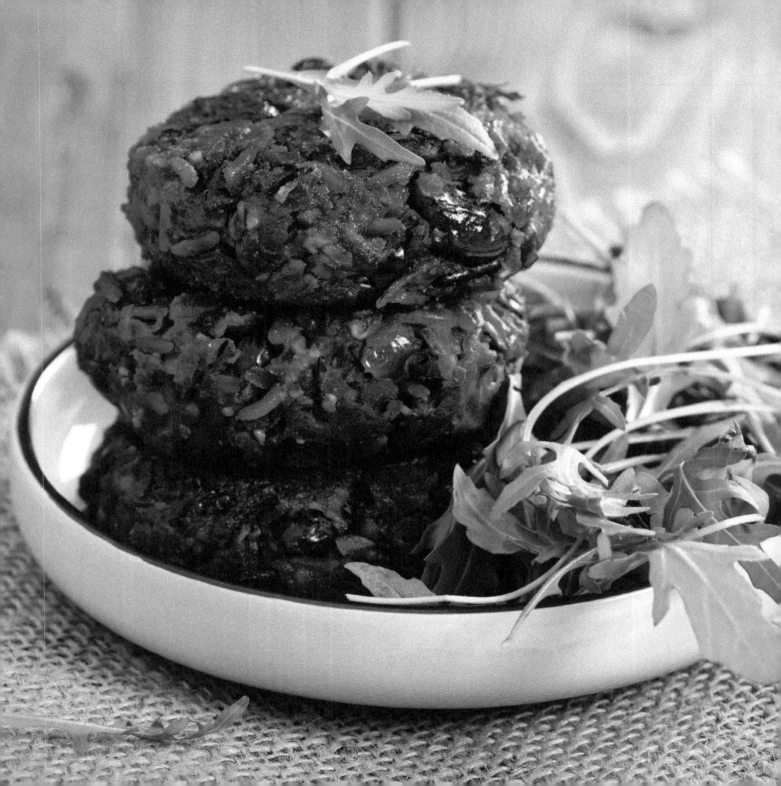

2. Ruby Red Root Beet Burger

Serves: 6 | Prep Time: ~20 min |

Nutrition Information
(per serving without buns)
- Calories: 159 kcal
- Carbs: 23.2 g.
- Fat: 4.9 g.
- Protein: 5.6 g.
- Fiber: 5.5 g.
- Sugar: 3.1 g.

INGREDIENTS:
- 3 cup chickpeas (canned or cooked)
- ½ cup dry quinoa
- 2 large beets
- 2 tbsp. olive oil
- 2 tbsp. garlic powder
- 1 tbsp. balsamic vinegar
- 2 tsp. onion powder
- 1 tsp. fresh parsley (chopped)
- Salt and pepper to taste
- 2 cups spinach (fresh or frozen, washed and dried)
- Optional: 6 buns or wraps of choice
- Optional: sauce of choice

Total number of ingredients: 13

METHOD:
1. Preheat the oven to 400°F / 200°C .
2. Prepare 1 cup of dry chickpeas according to the method on page 31.
3. Cook the quinoa according to the method on page 38.
4. Peel and dice the beets into ¼-inch or smaller cubes, put them in a bowl, and coat the cubes with 1 tablespoon of olive oil and the onion powder.
5. Spread the beet cubes out across a baking pan and put the pan in the oven.
6. Roast the beets until they have softened, approximately 10-15 minutes. Take them out and set aside so the beets can cool down.
7. After the beets have cooled down, transfer them into a food processor and add the cooked chickpeas and quinoa, vinegar, garlic, parsley, and a pinch of pepper and salt.
8. Pulse the ingredients until everything is crumbly, around 30 seconds.
9. Use your palms to form the mixture into 6 equal-sized patties and place them in a small pan.
10. Put them in a freezer, up to 1 hour, until the patties feel firm to the touch.
11. Heat up the remaining 1 tablespoon of olive oil in a skillet over medium-high heat and add the patties.
12. Cook them until they're browned on each side, about 4-6 minutes per side.
13. Store or serve the burgers with a handful of spinach, and if desired, on the bottom of the optional bun.
14. Top the burger with your sauce of choice.

STORAGE INFORMATION:

Storage	Temperature	Expiration date	Preparation
Airtight container M/L	Fridge at 38 – 40°F or 3°C	4-5 days after preparation	Reheat in pan or microwave
Airtight container M/L	Freezer at -1°F or -20°C	60 days after preparation	Thaw at room temperature; Reheat in pan or microwave

Note: Top these burgers with mustard, tahini, or vegan ranch!

Tip: Process the mixture until combined and crumbly. Be careful not to turn the ingredients into a paste or dough; this would mean the mixture is over-processed.

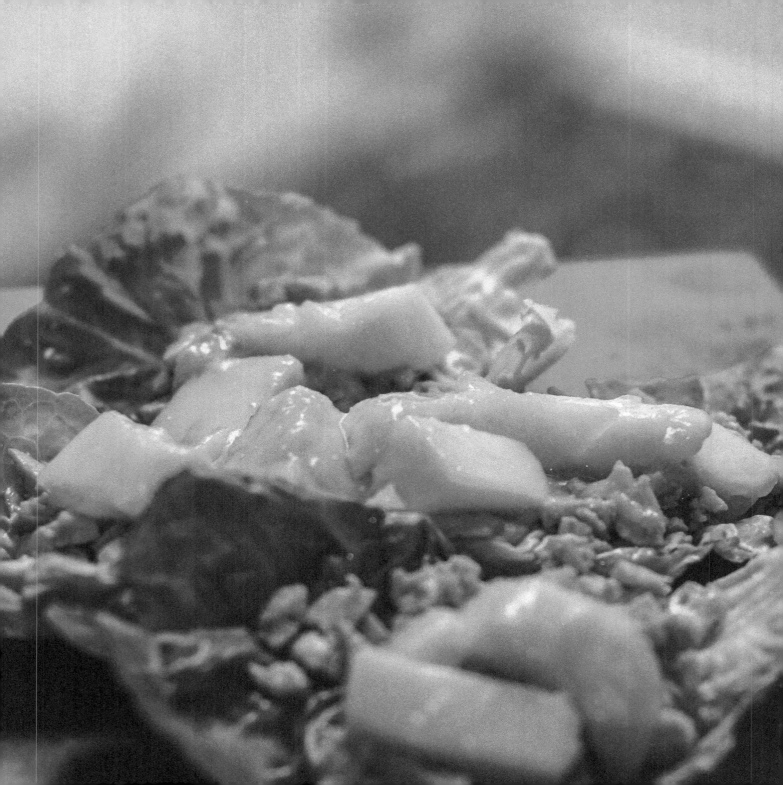

3. Mango-Tempeh Wraps

Nutrition Information
(per serving)
- Calories: 259 kcal
- Carbs: 31.3 g.
- Fat: 7.8 g.
- Protein: 15.7 g.
- Fiber: 9.7 g.
- Sugar: 16 g.

INGREDIENTS:

- **2 8-oz. blocks tempeh (drained, crumbled)**
- **1 tbsp. coconut oil**
- **6 large lettuce leaves**
- **2 medium ripe mangoes (peeled, diced)**
- **¼ cup sweet chili sauce**
- **1 tbsp. hoisin sauce**
- **1 tbsp. garlic powder**
- **¼ tsp. lime juice**
- **¼ tsp. salt**

Total number of ingredients: 9

METHOD:

1. Heat the coconut oil in a large skillet over medium heat.
2. Cook the tempeh crumbles until browned, stirring constantly, for about 4 minutes and turn the heat down to low.
3. Add the hoisin, garlic, salt, and lime juice; heat for an additional 2 minutes and set aside.
4. Cut the mangoes into ¼-inch cubes. Pour the sweet chili sauce into a small bowl and mix it with the mango cubes.
5. Scoop the cooked tempeh and divide it evenly between the lettuce leaves, using the leaves as wraps.
6. Top the wraps with the chunks of mango and a bit of lime juice and close the wraps.
7. Serve, share, or store!

STORAGE INFORMATION:

Storage	Temperature	Expiration date	Preparation
Airtight container M/L or Ziploc bag	Fridge at 38 – 40°F or 3°C	4-5 days after preparation	Eat chilled or reheat 10 seconds in the microwave
Airtight container M/L or Ziploc bag	Freezer at -1°F or -20°C	60 days after preparation	Thaw at room temperature; Eat chilled or reheat 10 seconds in the microwave

Note: Store the wraps already prepared, or, use multiple containers for the separate ingredients (tempeh, mangoes, and lettuce leaves).

4. Creamy Squash Pizza

Serves: 4 | Prep Time: ~25 min |

Nutrition Information
(per serving)
- Calories: 401 kcal
- Protein: 18.4 g.
- Fiber: 15.2 g.
- Carbs: 62.5 g.
- Sugar: 8.8 g.
- Fat: 8.6 g.

INGREDIENTS:

Sauce:
- 3 cups butternut squash (fresh or frozen, cubed)
- 2 tbsp. minced garlic
- 1 tbsp. olive oil
- 1 tsp. red pepper flakes
- 1 tsp. cumin
- 1 tsp. paprika
- 1 tsp. oregano

Crust:
- 2 cups dry French green lentils
- 2 cups water
- 2 tbsp. minced garlic
- 1 tbsp. Italian seasoning
- 1 tsp. onion powder

Toppings:
- 1 tbsp. olive oil
- 1 medium green bell pepper (pitted, diced)
- 1 medium red bell pepper (pitted, diced)
- 1 small head of broccoli (diced)
- 1 small purple onion (diced)

Total number of ingredients: 15

METHOD:

1. Preheat the oven to 350°F / 175°C.
2. Prepare the French green lentils according to the method on page 31.
3. Add all the sauce ingredients to a food processor or blender, and blend on low until everything has mixed and the sauce looks creamy. Set the sauce aside in a small bowl.
4. Clean the food processor or blender; then add all the ingredients for the crust and pulse on high speed until a dough-like batter has formed.
5. Heat a large deep-dish pan over medium-low heat and lightly grease it with 1 tablespoon of olive oil.
6. Press the crust dough into the skillet until it resembles a round pizza crust and cook until the crust is golden brown—about 5-6 minutes on each side.
7. Put the crust on a baking tray covered with parchment paper.
8. Coat the topside of the crust with the sauce using a spoon, and evenly distribute the toppings across the pizza.
9. Bake the pizza in the oven until the vegetables are tender and browned, for about 15 minutes.
10. Slice into 4 equal pieces and serve, or store.

STORAGE INFORMATION:

Storage	Temperature	Expiration date	Preparation
Airtight container S/M or Ziploc bag	Fridge at 38 – 40°F or 3°C	4-5 days after preparation	Reheat in the microwave
Airtight container S/M or Ziploc bag	Freezer at -1°F or -20°C	60 days after preparation	Thaw at room temperature. Reheat in the microwave

Note: Top this pizza with extra toppings or other vegetables.

Tip: Use a large skillet and press the crust out as flatly as possible. This way, the crust cooks quicker.

5. Lasagna Fungo

Nutrition Information
(per serving)
- Calories: 292 kcal
- Carbs: 38 g.
- Fat: 9.2 g.
- Protein:14.2 g.
- Fiber: 6.3 g.
- Sugar: 4.9 g.

INGREDIENTS:

- 10 lasagna noodles or sheets
- 2 cups matchstick carrots
- 1 cup mushrooms (sliced)
- 2 cups raw kale
- 1 14-oz. package extra firm tofu (drained)
- 1 cup hummus (pre-made or page 56)
- ½ cup nutritional yeast
- 2 tbsp. Italian seasoning
- 1 tbsp. garlic powder (or fresh, minced)
- 1 tbsp. olive oil
- 4 cups marinara sauce (page 185)
- 1 tsp. salt

Total number of ingredients: 12

METHOD:

1. Preheat the oven to 400°F / 200°C.
2. Cook the lasagna noodles or sheets according to the package instructions.
3. Take a large frying pan, put it over medium heat, and add the olive oil.
4. Throw in the carrots, mushrooms, and half a teaspoon of salt; cook for 5 minutes.
5. Add the kale, sauté for another 3 minutes, and remove the pan from the heat.
6. Take a large bowl, crumble in the tofu, and set the bowl aside for now.
7. Take another bowl and add the hummus, nutritional yeast, Italian seasoning, garlic, and ½ teaspoon salt; mix everything together.
8. Coat the bottom of an 8x8 baking dish with 1 cup of the marinara sauce.
9. Cover the sauce with a couple of the noodles or sheets, and top these with the tofu crumbles.
10. Add a layer of the vegetables and a tablespoon of hummus on top of the tofu.
11. Continue to build up the lasagna by stacking layers of marinara sauce, noodles or sheets, tofu, vegetables and hummus, and top it off with the remaining hummus.
12. Cover the lasagna with aluminum foil and bake in the oven for 20-25 minutes.
13. Remove the foil and put back in the oven for an additional 5 minutes.
14. Allow the lasagna to sit for 10 minutes before serving, or store for another day!

STORAGE INFORMATION:

Storage	Temperature	Expiration date	Preparation
Airtight container M/L	Fridge at 38 – 40°F or 3°C	4-5 days after preparation	Reheat in pot or microwave
Airtight container M/L	Freezer at -1°F or -20°C	60 days after preparation	Thaw at room temperature; Reheat in pot or microwave

Note: Top this lasagna with some vegan cheese before the last 5 minutes of baking for an ooey, gooey dish.

Tip: You can replace the lasagna noodles or sheets with sliced eggplant for a lower carb count and different flavor!

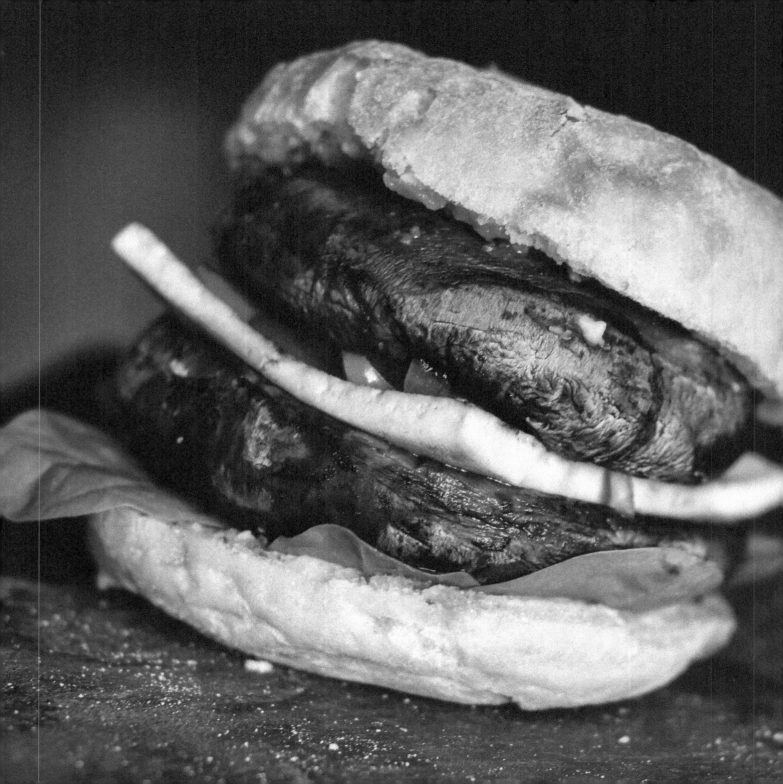

6. Stacked N' Spicy Portobello Burgers

Serves: 2 | Prep Time: ~30 min |

Nutrition Information
(per serving without bun)
- Calories: 421 kcal
- Carbs: 48.9 g.
- Fat: 16 g.
- Protein: 20.5 g.
- Fiber: 9.8 g.
- Sugar: 10.6 g.

INGREDIENTS:
- 1 8-oz. block firm tofu (drained)
- 1 tbsp. extra virgin olive oil
- 4 large portobello mushroom caps (stems removed)
- 1 large onion (diced)
- ½ green bell pepper (pitted, diced)
- ½ red bell pepper (pitted, diced)
- 3 cups spinach (fresh, rinsed, dried)
- 2 whole wheat vegan buns
- 4 tbsp. hummus (pre-made or page 56)
- ¼ cup salsa (page 187)
- 1 tbsp. taco seasoning
- ½ tsp. paprika
- ¼ tsp. chili powder
- Salt to taste

Total number of ingredients: 14

METHOD:
1. Cut the tofu into 4 large slices and set aside.
2. Heat the olive oil in a large skillet over medium-high heat.
3. Add the mushroom caps and flip them over after 4 minutes of cooking.
4. Sprinkle the caps with the taco seasoning, paprika, chili powder, and salt.
5. Flip again after 4 minutes, allowing them to cook until they have halved in size. Remove the caps from the skillet and set aside.
6. Add the tofu slices to the previously used skillet and cook them on both sides until slightly brown; set them aside.
7. Add the diced onions and bell peppers to the skillet. Stir frequently and cook the vegetables until browned, for 10-12 minutes.
8. Turn the heat down to low, add the mushrooms back to the skillet, and reheat for 2 more minutes.
9. Spread hummus on one side of each bun, and the salsa on the other half.
10. Top the hummus with a handful of spinach and serve with two mushroom caps, tofu squares, and top with a heaping scoop of vegetables with more salt to taste.
11. Enjoy the portobello burgers right away, or store and serve later!

Note: A thick slice of juicy tomato will really make these burgers pop! For storing, use a container for all the heated ingredients and a Ziploc bag for the buns or wraps.

Tip: Press down on the Portobello caps with a wooden spoon to remove the excess water faster.

STORAGE INFORMATION:

Storage	Temperature	Expiration date	Preparation
Airtight container M/L and Ziploc bag	Fridge at 38 – 40°F or 3°C	2-3 days after preparation	
Airtight container M/L and Ziploc bag	Freezer at -1°F or -20°C	60 days after preparation	Thaw at room temperature

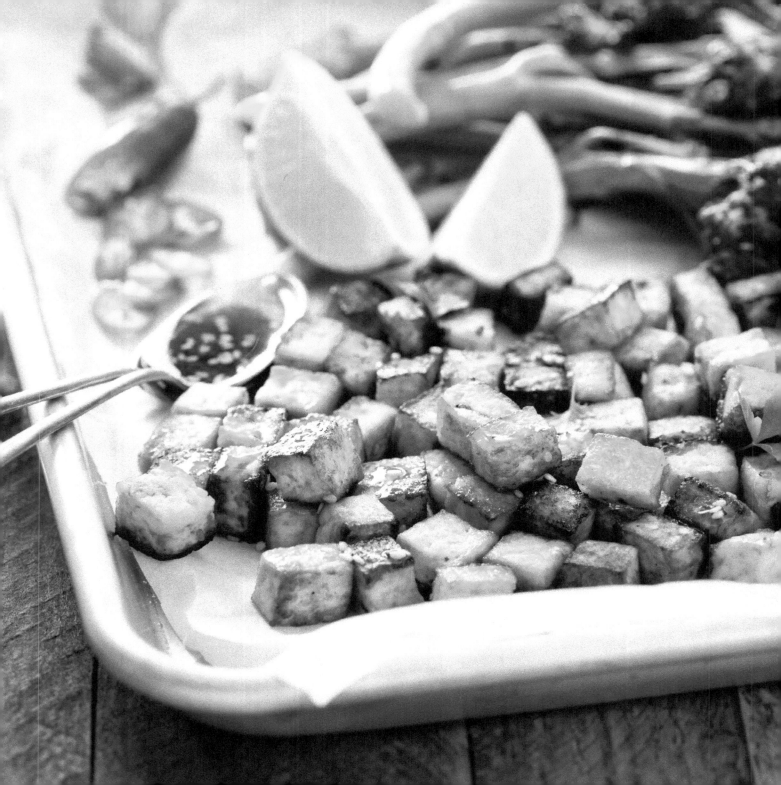

7. Sweet and Sour Tofu

Nutrition Information
(per serving)
- Calories: 236 kcal
- Carbs: 24.3 g.
- Fat: 11.5 g.
- Protein: 8.8 g.
- Fiber: 4.7 g.
- Sugar: 13.3 g.

INGREDIENTS:

- 1 14-oz. package extra firm tofu (drained)
- 2 tbsp. olive oil
- 1 large red bell pepper (pitted, chopped)
- 1 large green bell pepper (pitted, chopped)
- 1 medium white onion (diced)
- 2 tbsp. minced garlic
- ½-inch minced ginger
- 1 cup pineapple chunks
- 1 tbsp. tomato paste
- 2 tbsp. rice vinegar
- 2 tbsp. low sodium soy sauce
- 1 tsp. cornstarch
- 1 tbsp. coconut or cane sugar
- Salt and pepper to taste

Total number of ingredients: 15

METHOD:

1. In a small bowl, whisk together the tomato paste, vinegar, soy sauce, cornstarch, and sugar.
2. Cut the tofu into ¼-inch cubes, place in a medium bowl, and marinate in the soy sauce mixture until the tofu has absorbed the flavors (up to 3 hours).
3. Heat 1 tablespoon of the olive oil in a frying pan over medium-high heat.
4. Add the tofu chunks and half of the remaining marinade to the pan, leaving the rest for later.
5. Stir frequently until the tofu is cooked golden brown, approximately 10-12 minutes. Remove the tofu from the heat and set aside in a medium-sized bowl.
6. Add the other tablespoon of olive oil to the same pan, then the garlic and ginger; heat for about 1 minute.
7. Add in the peppers and onions. Stir until the vegetables have softened, about 5 minutes.
8. Pour the leftover marinade into the pan with the vegetables and heat until the sauce thickens while continuously stirring, around 4 minutes.
9. Add the pineapple chunks and tofu cubes to the pan while stirring and continue to cook for 3 minutes.
10. Serve and enjoy right away, or, let the sweet and sour tofu cool down and store for later!

Note: Marinate the tofu beforehand to reduce the prep time. This can be done overnight in a covered refrigerated bowl.

Tip: Serve over quinoa or rice for a more nutritious meal.

STORAGE INFORMATION:

Storage	Temperature	Expiration date	Preparation
Airtight container M/L	Fridge at 38 – 40°F or 3°C	3-4 days after preparation	Reheat in pot or microwave
Airtight container M/L	Freezer at -1°F or -20°C	60 days after preparation	Thaw at room temperature; Reheat on stove or in microwave

8. Stuffed Sweet Potatoes

Nutrition Information
(per serving)
- Calories: 498 kcal
- Carbs: 55.7 g.
- Fat: 17.1 g.
- Protein: 20.7 g.
- Fiber: 19.1 g.
- Sugar: 10.6 g.

INGREDIENTS:
- 1½ cup black beans (canned or cooked)
- 3 small or medium sweet potatoes
- 2 tbsp. olive oil
- 1 large red bell pepper (pitted, chopped)
- 1 large green bell pepper (pitted, chopped)
- 1 small sweet yellow onion (chopped)
- 2 tbsp. garlic (minced or powdered)
- 1 8-oz. package tempeh (diced into ¼" cubes)
- ½ cup marinara sauce (page 185)
- ½ cup water
- 1 tbsp. chili powder
- 1 tsp. parsley
- ½ tsp. cayenne
- Salt and pepper to taste

Total number of ingredients: 15

METHOD:
1. Preheat the oven to 400°F / 200°C.
2. When using dry beans, prepare ½ cup of dry black beans according to the method on page 31.
3. Using a fork, poke several holes in the skins of the sweet potatoes.
4. Wrap the sweet potatoes tightly with aluminum foil and place them in the oven until soft and tender, or for approximately 45 minutes.
5. While sweet potatoes are cooking, heat the olive oil in a deep pan over medium-high heat. Add the onions, bell peppers, and garlic; cook until the onions are tender, for about 10 minutes.
6. Add the water, together with the cooked beans, marinara sauce, chili powder, parsley, and cayenne. Bring the mixture to a boil and then lower the heat to medium or low. Allow the mixture to simmer until the liquid has thickened, for about 15 minutes.
7. Add the diced tempeh cubes and heat until warmed, around 1 minute.
8. Blend in salt and pepper to taste.
9. When the potatoes are done baking, remove them from the oven. Cut a slit across the top of each one, but do not split the potatoes all the way in half.
10. Top each potato with a scoop of the beans, vegetables, and tempeh mixture. Place the filled potatoes back in the hot oven for about 5 minutes.
11. Serve after cooling for a few minutes, or, store for another day!

STORAGE INFORMATION:

Storage	Temperature	Expiration date	Preparation
2-compartment airtight container M/L	Fridge at 38 – 40°F or 3°C	4-5 days after preparation	Reheat in pot or microwave
2-compartment airtight container M/L	Freezer at -1°F or -20°C	60 days after preparation	Thaw at room temperature; Reheat in pot or microwave

Note: You can replace the sweet potatoes with bell peppers, squash, eggplants, and more! The possibilities are endless but note that the oven time may differ.

Tip: If the filling seems too thick, add a tablespoon of water. If it seems too runny, add a touch of cornstarch to thicken.

9. Satay Tempeh with Cauliflower Rice

Serves: 4 | Prep Time: ~60 min |

Nutrition Information
(per serving)
- Calories: 531 kcal
- Carbs: 31.7 g.
- Fat: 33 g.
- Protein: 27.6 g.
- Fiber: 14.8 g.
- Sugar: 10.4 g.

INGREDIENTS:

Sauce:

- ¼ cup water
- 4 tbsp. peanut butter
  (page 43)
- 3 tbsp. low sodium soy sauce
- 2 tbsp. coconut sugar
- 1 garlic clove (minced)
- ½-inch ginger (minced)
- 2 tsp. rice vinegar
- 1 tsp. red pepper flakes

Main ingredients:

- 4 tbsp. olive oil
- 2 8-oz. packages tempeh
  (drained)
- 2 cups cauliflower rice
- 1 cup purple cabbage (diced)
- 1 tbsp. sesame oil
- 1 tsp. agave nectar

Total number of ingredients: 14

METHOD:

1. Take a large bowl, combine all the ingredients for the sauce, and then whisk until the mixture is smooth and any lumps have dissolved.
2. Cut the tempeh into ½-inch cubes and put them into the sauce, stirring to make sure the cubes get coated thoroughly.
3. Place the bowl in the refrigerator to marinate the tempeh for up to 3 hours.
4. Before the tempeh is done marinating, preheat the oven to 400°F / 200°C.
5. Spread the tempeh out in a single layer on a baking sheet lined with parchment paper or lightly greased with olive oil.
6. Bake the marinated cubes until browned and crisp—about 15 minutes.
7. Heat the cauliflower rice in a saucepan with 2 tablespoons of olive oil over medium heat until it is warm.
8. Rinse the large bowl with water, and then mix the cabbage, sesame oil, and agave together.
9. Serve a scoop of the cauliflower rice topped with the marinated cabbage and cooked tempeh on a plate or in a bowl and enjoy. Or, store for later.

STORAGE INFORMATION:

Storage	Temperature	Expiration date	Preparation
3-compart-ment airtight container M/L	Fridge at 38 – 40°F or 3°C	4-5 days after preparation	Reheat in pot or microwave
3-compart-ment airtight container M/L	Freezer at -1°F or -20°C	60 days after preparation	Thaw at room temperature; Reheat in pot or microwave

Note: Sesame seeds make a great garnish! Store the cauliflower rice, cabbage, and tempeh in a 3-compartment container or separate containers.

Tip: Use a food processor to make rice from a head of fresh cauliflower.

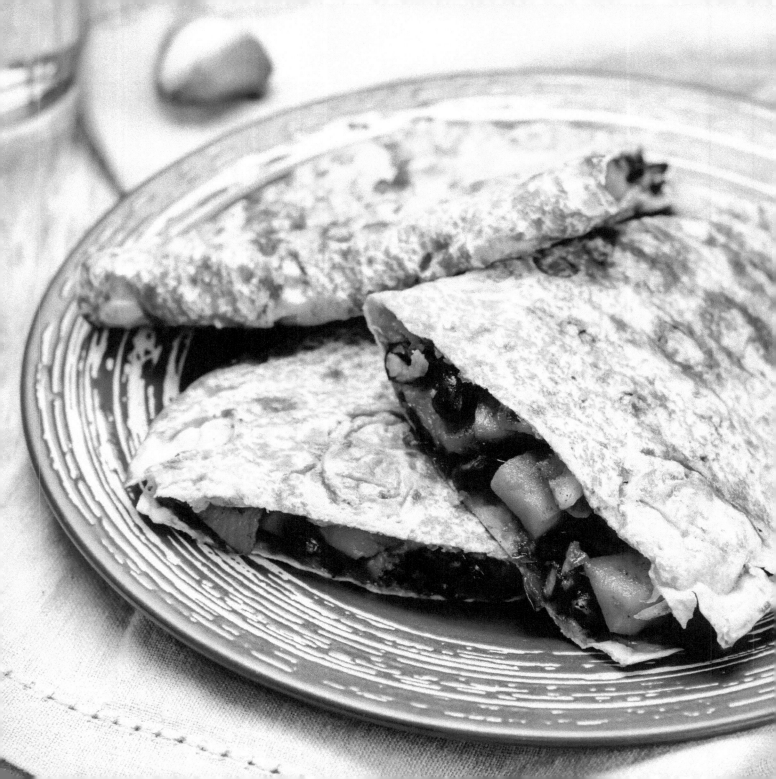

10. Sweet Potato Quesadillas

Nutrition Information
(per serving)
- Calories: 329 kcal
- Carbs: 54.8 g.
- Fat: 7.5 g.
- Protein: 10.6 g.
- Fiber: 8.3 g.
- Sugar: 3.1 g.

INGREDIENTS:

- **3 cups black beans (canned or cooked)**
- **½ cup dry brown rice**
- **1 large sweet potato (peeled and diced)**
- **½ cup salsa (page 187)**
- **3-6 tortilla wraps (page 55)**
- **1 tbsp. olive oil**
- **½ tsp. garlic powder**
- **½ tsp. onion powder**
- **½ tsp. paprika**

Total number of ingredients: 9

METHOD:

1. Preheat the oven to 350°F / 175°C.
2. When using dry beans, prepare 1 cup of dry black beans according to the method on page 31.
3. Cook the brown rice according to the method on page 37.
4. Line a baking pan with parchment paper.
5. Cut the sweet potato into ½-inch cubes and drizzle these with olive oil. Transfer the cubes to the baking pan.
6. Place the pan in the oven and bake the potatoes until tender, for around 1 hour.
7. Allow the potatoes to cool for 5 minutes and then add them to a large mixing bowl with the salsa and cooked rice. Use a fork to mash the ingredients together into a thoroughly combined mixture.
8. Heat a saucepan over medium-high heat and add the potato/rice mixture, cooked black beans, and spices to the pan.
9. Cook everything for about 5 minutes or until it is heated through.
10. Take another frying pan and put it over medium-low heat. Place a tortilla in the pan and fill half of it with a heaping scoop of the potato, bean, and rice mixture.
11. Fold the tortilla in half to cover the filling and cook the tortilla until both sides are browned—about 4 minutes per side.
12. Serve the tortillas with some additional salsa on the side.

STORAGE INFORMATION:

Storage	Temperature	Expiration date	Preparation
2-compartment airtight container M/L	Fridge at 38 – 40°F or 3°C	4-5 days after preparation	Reheat in pan or microwave
2-compartment airtight container M/L	Freezer at -1°F or -20°C	60 days after preparation	Thaw at room temperature; Reheat in pan or microwave

Note: Don't overstuff the tortilla to avoid having trouble flipping it. Stick to around half a cup of filling or slightly less.

Tip: Feel free to top the tortillas with vegan cheese, jalapeños, and/or fresh cubed tomatoes.

11. Teriyaki Tofu Wraps

Nutrition Information
(per serving)
- Calories: 259 kcal
- Carbs: 20.5 g.
- Fat: 15.4 g.
- Protein: 12.1 g.
- Fiber: 3.2 g.
- Sugar: 11.6 g.

INGREDIENTS:
- 1 14-oz. package extra firm tofu (drained)
- 1 small white onion (diced)
- ½ pineapple (peeled, cored)
- ¼ cup soy sauce
- 2 tbsp. sesame oil
- 1 garlic clove (minced, or ½ tsp. garlic powder)
- 1 tbsp. coconut sugar
- 3-6 large lettuce leaves
- 1 tbsp. roasted sesame seeds
- Salt and pepper to taste

Total number of ingredients: 11

METHOD:
1. Take a medium-sized bowl and mix the soy sauce, sesame oil, coconut sugar, and garlic.
2. Cut the tofu into ½-inch cubes, place them in the bowl, and transfer the bowl to the refrigerator to marinate, up to 3 hours.
3. Meanwhile, cut the pineapple into rings or cubes.
4. After the tofu is adequately marinated, place a large skillet over medium heat, and pour in the tofu with the remaining marinade, pineapple cubes, and diced onions; stir.
5. Add salt and pepper to taste, making sure to stir the ingredients frequently, and cook until the onions are soft and translucent—about 15 minutes.
6. Divide the mixture between the lettuce leaves and top with a sprinkle of roasted sesame seeds.
7. Serve right away, or, store the mixture and lettuce leaves separately.

STORAGE INFORMATION:

Storage	Temperature	Expiration date	Preparation
2-compartment airtight container M	Fridge at 38 – 40°F or 3°C	4-5 days after preparation	Reheat in pot or microwave
2-compartment airtight container M	Freezer at -1°F or -20°C	60 days after preparation	Thaw at room temperature; Reheat in pot or microwave

Note: Butter, Bibb and Iceberg lettuce leaves work best for these wraps.

Tip: Replace the soy sauce with tamari for a different taste and a gluten-free dish.

12. Tex-Mex Tofu & Beans

Serves: 4 | Prep Time: ~25 min |

Nutrition Information
(per serving)
- Calories: 315 kcal
- Carbs: 27.8 g.
- Fat: 17 g.
- Protein: 12.7 g.
- Fiber: 7.5 g.
- Sugar: 1.9 g.

INGREDIENTS:
- **3 cups black beans (canned or cooked)**
- **1 cup dry brown rice**
- **1 14-oz. package firm tofu (drained)**
- **2 tbsp. olive oil**
- **1 small purple onion (diced)**
- **1 medium avocado (pitted, peeled)**
- **1 garlic clove (minced)**
- **1 tbsp. lime juice**
- **2 tsp. cumin**
- **2 tsp. paprika**
- **1 tsp. chili powder**
- **Salt and pepper to taste**

Total number of ingredients: 13

METHOD:

1. When using dry beans, prepare 1 cup of dry black beans according to the method on page 31.
2. Cook the rice according to the method on page 37.
3. Cut the tofu into ½-inch cubes.
4. Heat the olive oil in a large skillet over high heat. Add the diced onions and cook until soft, for about 5 minutes.
5. Add the tofu and cook an additional 2 minutes, flipping the cubes frequently.
6. Meanwhile, cut the avocado into thin slices and set aside.
7. Lower the heat to medium and mix in the garlic, cumin, and cooked black beans.
8. Stir until everything is incorporated thoroughly, and then cook for an additional 5 minutes.
9. Add the remaining spices and lime juice to the mixture in the skillet.
10. Mix thoroughly and remove the skillet from the heat.
11. Serve the Tex-Mex tofu and beans with a scoop of rice and garnish with the fresh avocado.
12. Enjoy immediately, or, store the rice, avocado, and tofu mixture separately.

STORAGE INFORMATION:

Storage	Temperature	Expiration date	Preparation
3-compartment airtight container M/L	Fridge at 38 – 40°F or 3°C	4-5 days after preparation	Reheat in pot or microwave
3-compartment airtight container M/L	Freezer at -1°F or -20°C	60 days after preparation	Thaw at room temperature; Reheat in pot or microwave

Note: Vegan ranch, sour cream, and/or jalapeños are also great toppings!

Tip: Press the water out of the tofu before cooking. This will reduce the time it needs to brown.

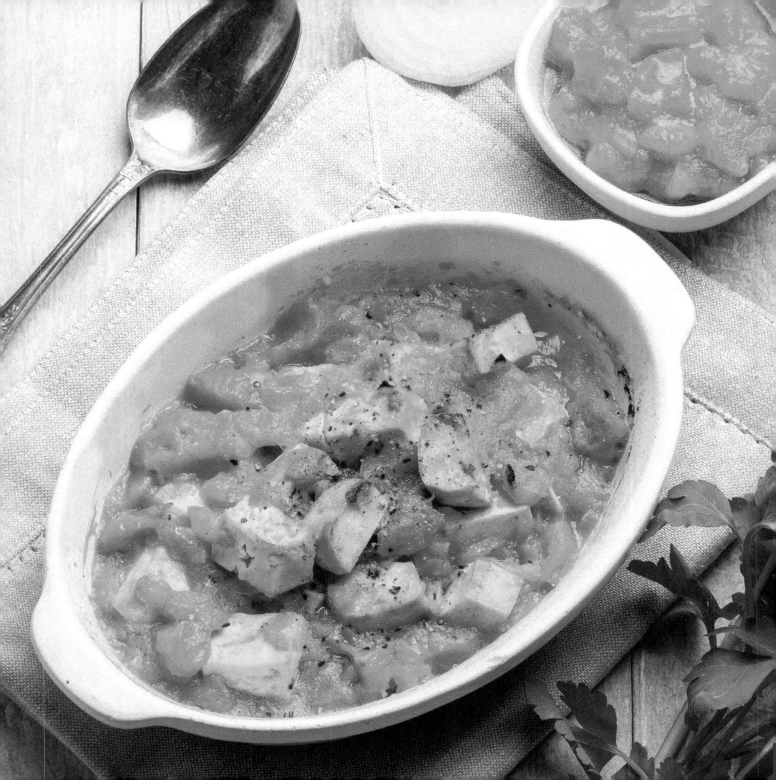

13. Tofu Cacciatore

Serves: 3 | Prep Time: 45 min |

Nutrition Information
(per serving)
- Calories: 274 kcal
- Carbs: 33.7 g.
- Fat: 9.5 g.
- Protein: 13.6 g.
- Fiber: 7.3 g.
- Sugar: 14.9 g.

INGREDIENTS:

- 1 14-oz. package extra firm tofu (drained)
- 1 tbsp. olive oil
- 1 cup matchstick carrots
- 1 medium sweet onion (diced)
- 1 medium green bell pepper (seeded, diced)
- 1 28-oz. can diced tomatoes
- 1 4-oz. can tomato paste
- ½ tbsp. balsamic vinegar
- 1 tbsp. soy sauce
- 1 tbsp. maple syrup
- 1 tbsp. garlic powder (or fresh, minced)
- 1 tbsp. Italian seasoning
- Salt and pepper to taste

Total number of ingredients: 14

METHOD:

1. Chop the tofu into ¼- to ½-inch cubes.
2. Heat the olive oil in a large skillet over medium-high heat.
3. Add the onions, garlic, bell peppers, and carrots; sauté until the onions turn translucent, around 10 minutes. Make sure to stir frequently to prevent burning.
4. Now add the balsamic vinegar, soy sauce, maple syrup, garlic powder and Italian seasoning.
5. Stir well while pouring in the diced tomatoes and tomato paste; mix until all ingredients are thoroughly combined.
6. Add the cubed tofu and stir one more time.
7. Cover the pot, turn the heat to medium-low, and allow the mixture to simmer until the sauce has thickened, for around 20-25 minutes.
8. Serve the tofu cacciatore in bowls and top with salt and pepper to taste, or, store for another meal!

STORAGE INFORMATION:

Storage	Temperature	Expiration date	Preparation
Airtight container M/L	Fridge at 38 – 40°F or 3°C	5-6 days after preparation	Reheat in pot or microwave
Airtight container M/L	Freezer at -1°F or -20°C	60 days after preparation	Thaw at room temperature; Reheat on the stove or microwave

Note: You can add more veggies to the mix, such as red bell peppers, fresh tomatoes, zucchini, and/or squash!

Tip: If the sauce tastes too acidic, add more maple syrup. If the sauce is too sweet, add another dollop of tomato paste.

14. Vegan Friendly Fajitas

Serves: 6 | Prep Time: ~30 min |

Nutrition Information
(per serving)
- Calories: 264 kcal
- Carbs: 27.7 g.
- Fat: 14 g.
- Protein: 6.8 g.
- Fiber: 7.6 g.
- Sugar: 4.3 g.

INGREDIENTS:
- 3 cups black beans (canned or cooked)
- 1 large green bell pepper (seeded, diced)
- 1 poblano pepper (seeded, thinly sliced)
- 1 large avocado (peeled, pitted, mashed)
- 1 medium sweet onion (chopped)
- 3 large portobello mushrooms (stems removed and sliced)
- 2 tbsp. olive oil
- 6 tortilla wraps (page 55)
- 1 tsp. lime juice
- 1 tsp. chili powder
- 1 tsp. garlic powder
- ¼ tsp. cayenne pepper
- Salt to taste

Total number of ingredients: 13

METHOD:

1. When using dry beans, prepare 1 cup of dry black beans according to the method on page 31.
2. Heat 1 tablespoon of olive oil in a large frying pan over high heat.
3. Add the bell peppers, poblano peppers, and half of the onions.
4. Mix in the chili powder, garlic powder, and cayenne pepper; add salt to taste.
5. Cook the vegetables until tender and browned, around 10 minutes.
6. Add the black beans and continue cooking for an additional 2 minutes; then remove the frying pan from the stove.
7. Add the portobello mushrooms to the skillet and turn heat down to low. Sprinkle the mushrooms with salt.
8. Stir/flip the ingredients often and cook until the mushrooms have shrank down to half their size, around 7 minutes. Remove the frying pan from the heat.
9. Mix the avocado, remaining 1 tablespoon of olive oil, and the remaining onions together in a small bowl to make a simple guacamole. Mix in the lime juice and add salt and pepper to taste.
10. Spread the guacamole on a tortilla with a spoon and then top with a generous scoop of the mushroom mixture.
11. Serve and enjoy right away, or, allow the prepared tortillas to cool down and wrap them in paper towels to store!

STORAGE INFORMATION:

Storage	Temperature	Expiration date	Preparation
Airtight container M/L or Ziploc bag	Fridge at 38 – 40°F or 3°C	5-6 days after preparation	Remove paper towel and reheat in oven or microwave
Airtight container M/L or Ziploc bag	Freezer at -1°F or -20°C	60 days after preparation	Thaw at room temperature; Remove paper towel and reheat in oven or microwave

Note: Garnish the tortillas with finely chopped purple or sweet onions, salsa, vegan sour cream, and/or extra lime juice.

Tip: Make sure to remove all poblano seeds or the tortillas may be too spicy.

15. Portobello Burritos

Serves: 4 | Prep Time: ~50 min |

Nutrition Information
(per serving)
- Calories: 239 kcal
- Carbs: 34 g.
- Fat: 9.2 g.
- Protein: 5.1 g.
- Fiber: 7.4 g.
- Sugar: 6.8 g.

INGREDIENTS:

- **3 large portobello mushrooms (stems removed)**
- **2 medium potatoes**
- **4 tortilla wraps (page 55)**
- **1 medium avocado (pitted, peeled, diced)**
- **¾ cup salsa (page 187)**
- **1 tbsp. cilantro**
- **½ tsp. salt**

Marinade:
- **⅓ cup water**
- **1 tbsp. lime juice**
- **1 tbsp. minced garlic**
- **¼ cup teriyaki sauce**

Total number of ingredients: 11

METHOD:

1. Preheat the oven to 400°F / 200°C.
2. Lightly grease a sheet pan with olive oil (or alternatively, line with parchment paper) and set it aside.
3. Combine the water, lime juice, teriyaki, and garlic in a small bowl.
4. Slice the portobello mushrooms into thin slices and add these to the bowl. Allow the mushrooms to marinate thoroughly, for up to three hours.
5. Cut the potatoes into large matchsticks, like French fries. Sprinkle the fries with salt and then transfer them to the sheet pan. Place the fries in the oven and bake them until crisped and golden, around 30 minutes. Flip once halfway through for even cooking.
6. Heat a large frying pan over medium heat. Add the marinated mushroom slices with the remaining marinade to the pan. Cook until the liquid has absorbed, around 10 minutes. Remove from heat.
7. Fill the tortillas with a heaping scoop of the mushrooms and a handful of the potato sticks. Top with salsa, sliced avocados, and cilantro before serving.
8. Serve right away and enjoy, or, store the tortillas, avocado, and mushrooms separately for later!

STORAGE INFORMATION:

Storage	Temperature	Expiration date	Preparation
3-section airtight container M/L	Fridge at 38 – 40°F or 3°C	4-5 days after preparation	Reheat in stove or microwave
3-section airtight container M/L	Freezer at -1°F or -20°C	60 days after preparation	Thaw at room temperature; Reheat in the stove or microwave

Note: Add shredded vegan cheese, sour cream, more avocado, and/or guacamole to these burritos.

Tip: Marinate the mushrooms before cooking to save on prep time.

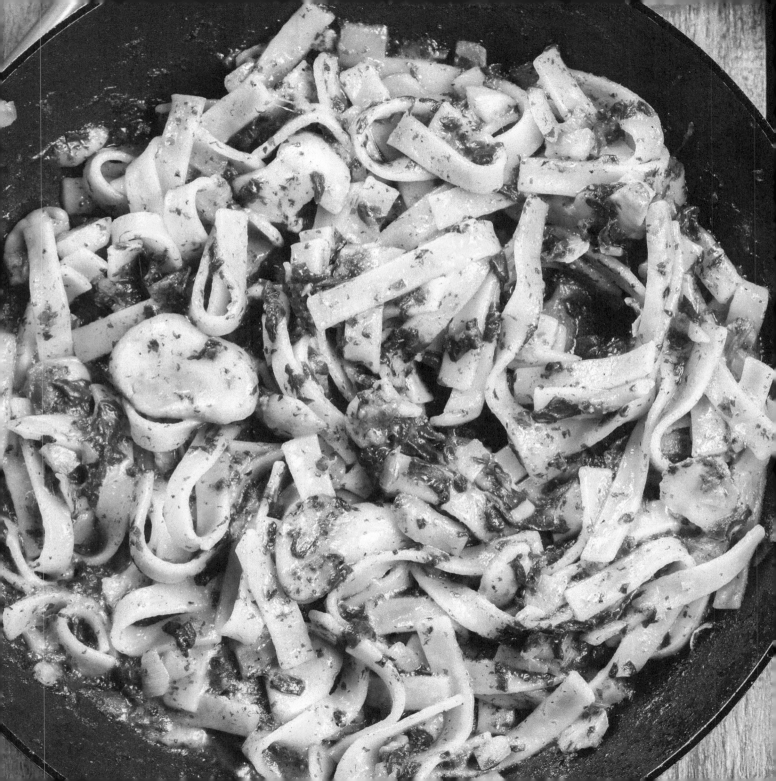

16. Mushroom Madness Stroganoff

Serves: 4 | Prep Time: ~30 min |

Nutrition Information
(per serving)
- Calories: 200 kcal
- Carbs: 27.8 g.
- Fat: 6.5 g.
- Protein: 7.6 g.
- Fiber: 4.9 g.
- Sugar: 2.2 g.

INGREDIENTS:
- **2 cups gluten-free noodles**
- **1 small onion (chopped)**
- **2 cups vegetable broth (page 49)**
- **2 tbsp. almond flour**
- **1 tbsp. tamari**
- **1 tsp. tomato paste**
- **1 tsp. lemon juice**
- **3 cups mushrooms (chopped)**
- **1 tsp. thyme**
- **3 cups raw spinach**
- **1 tbsp. apple cider vinegar**
- **1 tbsp. olive oil**
- **Salt and pepper to taste**
- **2 tbsp. fresh parsley (optional, diced)**

Total number of ingredients: 15

METHOD:
1. Prepare the noodles according to the package instructions.
2. Heat the olive oil in a large skillet over medium heat.
3. Add the chopped onion and sauté until soft—for about 5 minutes.
4. Stir in the flour, vegetable broth, tamari, tomato paste, and lemon juice; cook for an additional 3 minutes.
5. Blend in the mushrooms, thyme, and salt to taste, then cover the skillet.
6. Cook until the mushrooms are tender, for about 7 minutes, and turn the heat down to low.
7. Add the cooked noodles, spinach, and vinegar to the pan and top the ingredients with salt and pepper to taste.
8. Cover the skillet again and let the flavors combine for another 8-10 minutes.
9. Serve immediately, topped with the optional parsley if desired, or, store and enjoy the stroganoff another day of the week!

STORAGE INFORMATION:

Storage	Temperature	Expiration date	Preparation
Airtight container M/L	Fridge at 38 – 40°F or 3°C	3-4 days after preparation	Reheat in pot or microwave
Airtight container M/L	Freezer at -1°F or -20°C	60 days after preparation	Thaw at room temperature; Reheat in pot or microwave

Note: All kinds of mushrooms taste great in this recipe!

Tip: Mix in some vegan sour cream for a thicker stroganoff sauce.

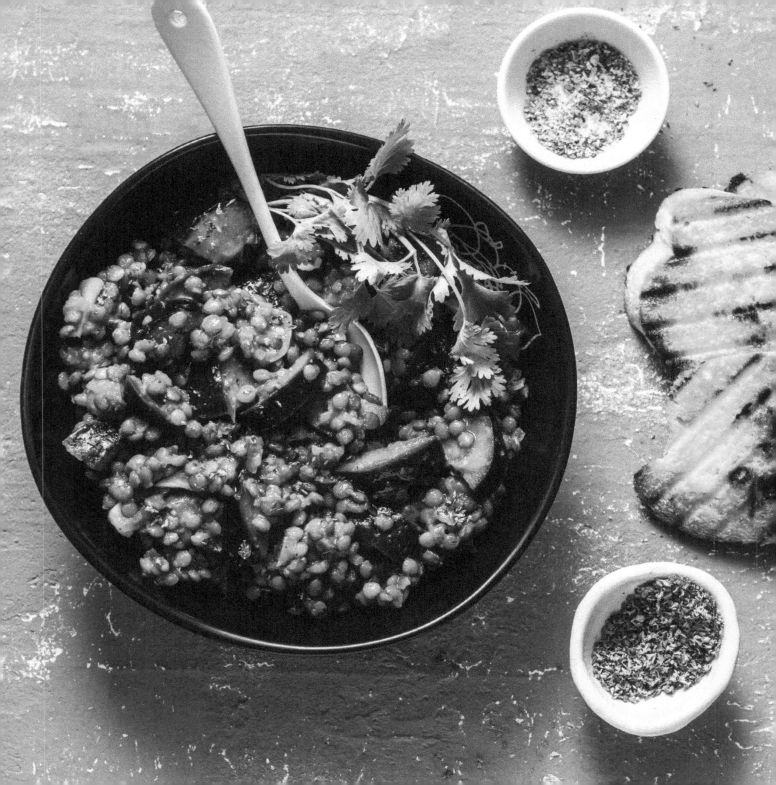

17. Moroccan Eggplant Stew

Nutrition Information
(per serving)
- Calories: 417 kcal
- Carbs: 80.5 g.
- Fat: 2.7 g.
- Protein: 17.7 g.
- Fiber: 23.9 g.
- Sugar: 26.5 g.

INGREDIENTS:

- **3 cups green lentils (canned or cooked)**
- **3 cups chickpeas (canned or cooked)**
- **1 tsp. olive oil**
- **1 large sweet onion (chopped)**
- **1 medium green bell pepper (seeded, diced)**
- **1 large eggplant**
- **1 cup vegetable broth (page 49)**
- **¾ cup tomato sauce**
- **½ cup golden raisins**
- **2 tbsp. turmeric**
- **1 garlic clove (minced)**
- **1 tsp. cumin**
- **½ tsp. allspice**
- **¼ tsp. chili powder**
- **Salt and pepper to taste**

Total number of ingredients: 16

METHOD:

1. When using dry lentils, prepare 1 cup of dry lentils according to the method on page 31.
2. When using dry chickpeas, prepare 1 cup of dry chickpeas according to the method on page 31.
3. Heat the olive oil in a medium-sized skillet over medium high heat.
4. Add the onions and cook until they begin to caramelize and soften, in 5-8 minutes.
5. Cut the eggplant into ½-inch eggplant cubes and add it to the skillet along with the bell pepper, cumin, allspice, garlic, and turmeric.
6. Stir the ingredients to combine everything evenly and heat for about 4 minutes; then add the vegetable broth and tomato sauce.
7. Cover the skillet, turn the heat down to low, and simmer the ingredients until the eggplant feels tender, or for about 20 minutes. You should be able to easily insert a fork into the cubes.
8. Uncover and mix in the cooked chickpeas and green lentils, as well as the raisins and chili powder. Simmer the ingredients until all the flavors have melded together, or for about 3 minutes.
9. Store the stew for later, or, serve in a bowl, top with salt and pepper to taste, and enjoy!

STORAGE INFORMATION:

Storage	Temperature	Expiration date	Preparation
Airtight container M/L	Fridge at 38 – 40°F or 3°C	4-5 days after preparation	Reheat in pot or microwave
Airtight container M/L	Freezer at -1°F or -20°C	60 days after preparation	Thaw at room temperature; Reheat in pot or microwave

Note: You can also substitute the green lentils with brown or red lentils if desired.

Tip: Be sure not to cut the eggplant too large or it may not cook thoroughly.

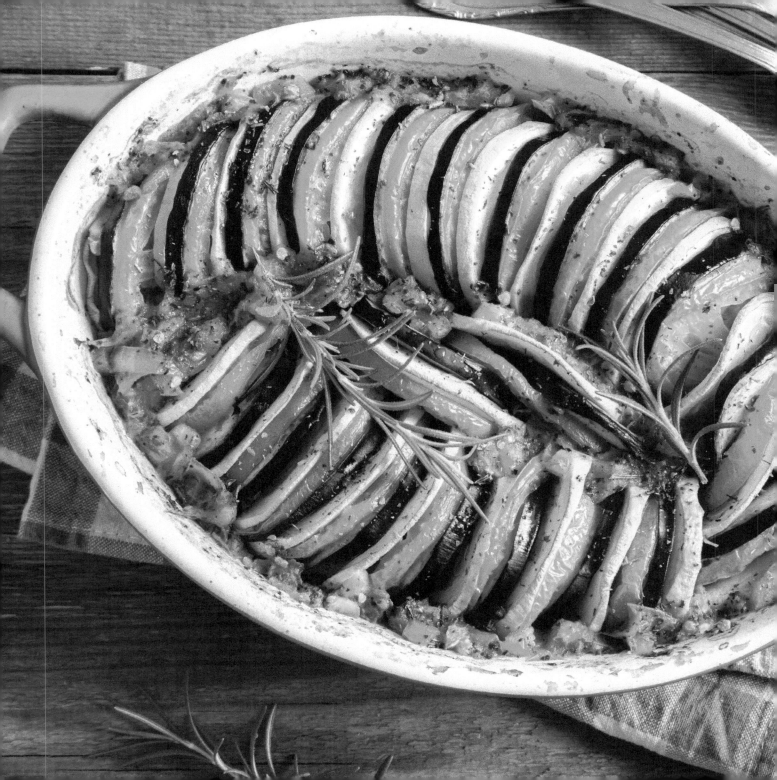

18. Refined Ratatouille

Nutrition Information
(per serving)
- Calories: 558 kcal
- Carbs: 61.2 g.
- Fat: 24.3 g.
- Protein: 23.7 g.
- Fiber: 19.1 g.
- Sugar: 31.6 g.

INGREDIENTS:
- 1 14-oz. block extra firm tofu (drained)
- 2 large heirloom tomatoes
- 1 large eggplant
- 1 large zucchini
- 1 large yellow squash
- 1 large sweet yellow onion (diced)
- 1 cup chopped kale
- 1 cup tomato sauce
- 2 tbsp. olive oil
- 1 tbsp. minced garlic
- ¼ tsp. chili powder
- ¼ tsp. apple cider vinegar
- ⅛ tsp. fennel seeds
- Salt and pepper to taste
- 5-6 large basil leaves (finely chopped)

Total number of ingredients: 16

METHOD:
1. Preheat the oven to 350°F / 175°C.
2. Lightly grease an 8x8" square dish with 1 tablespoon of olive oil and set it aside.
3. Combine the tomato sauce, vinegar, remaining 1 tablespoon of olive oil, garlic, fennel seeds, and chili powder in a large mixing bowl.
4. Add salt and pepper to taste and stir until all ingredients are evenly coated.
5. Pour the mixture into the baking dish and use a spoon to smear the ingredients out evenly across the bottom of the dish.
6. Lay out the kale in one even layer on top of the mixture.
7. Vertically slice the tomatoes, eggplant, zucchini, squash, and onion into thick, round discs; they should look like miniature plates or saucers.
8. Cut the tofu into thin slices, each similar in size to the vegetable discs for even cooking.
9. Layer the vegetable discs and tofu slices on top of the kale in the baking dish with an alternating pattern. For instance: tomato, eggplant, tofu, zucchini, squash, onion, repeat.
10. Fill up every inch of the pan with all the slices and stack them against the edge.
11. Place the baking dish into the oven and bake until the tomato sauce has thickened, and the vegetable slices have softened, around 50 minutes to an hour.
12. Scoop the ratatouille into a bowl and garnish it with the chopped basil.
13. Serve and enjoy, or, store for another day!

STORAGE INFORMATION:

Storage	Temperature	Expiration date	Preparation
Airtight container M/L	Fridge at 38 – 40°F or 3°C	3-4 days after preparation	Reheat in pot or microwave or serve chilled
Airtight container M/L	Freezer at -1°F or -20°C	60 days after preparation	Thaw at room temperature; Reheat in pot or microwave or serve chilled

Note: Experiment with using other vegetables—like bell pepper, shallots, or even potatoes—for a different flavor profile!

Tip: Use the freshest, most flavorful veggies since they're the real star of this dish. Extra firm tofu holds up better during the cooking process than softer blocks.

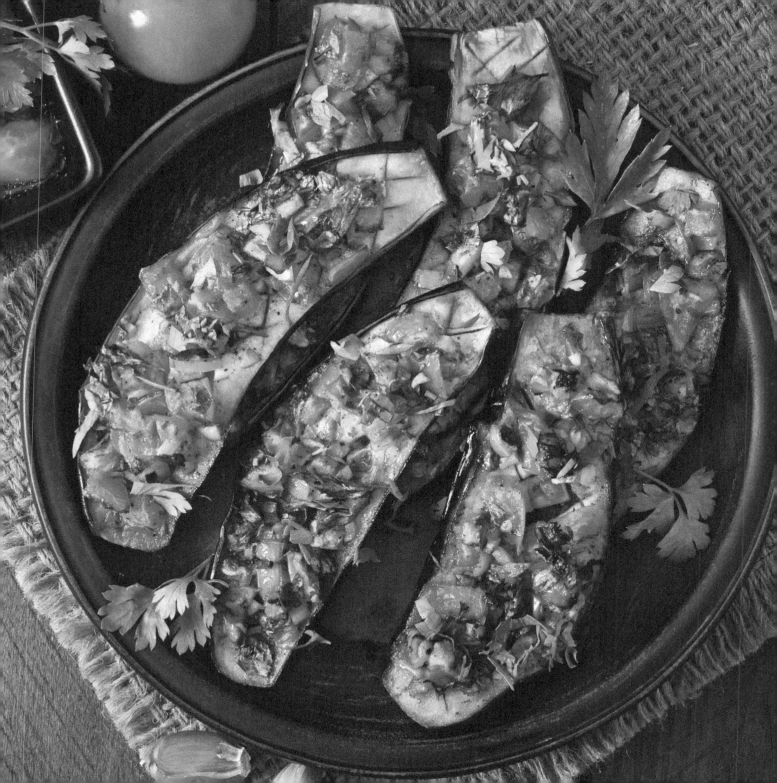

19. Stuffed Indian Eggplant

Nutrition Information
(per serving)
- Calories: 145 kcal
- Carbs: 18.3 g.
- Fat: 6 g.
- Protein: 4.4 g.
- Fiber: 6.6 g.
- Sugar: 8.1 g.

INGREDIENTS:
- 1½ cup black beans (canned or cooked)
- 6 medium eggplants (peeled)
- 3 large Roma tomatoes (diced)
- 1 large purple onion (chopped)
- 1 large yellow bell pepper (chopped)
- 2 cups raw spinach
- 2 tbsp. olive oil
- 2 cloves garlic (minced, or 1 tsp. powder)
- 1 tbsp. tomato paste
- 1 tsp. coconut sugar
- 1 tsp. cumin
- 1 tsp. turmeric
- Salt and pepper to taste
- 2 tbsp. thyme (optional, chopped)

Total number of ingredients: 15

METHOD:

1. When using dry beans, prepare ½ cup of dry black beans according to the method on page 31.
2. Preheat the oven to 400°F / 200°C.
3. Line a large baking sheet or pan with parchment paper and set it aside.
4. Cut the peeled eggplants open across the top from one side to the other, being careful not to slice all the way through.
5. Sprinkle the inside of the cut eggplants with salt and wrap them in a paper towel to drain the excess water. This could take up to 30 minutes.
6. Place the eggplants on the baking sheet and bake in the oven for 15 minutes. Remove the baking sheet from the oven and set it aside.
7. Heat 1 tablespoon of olive oil in a large skillet over medium-high heat. Add the chopped onions and sauté until soft, around 5 minutes.
8. Stir frequently, adding in the bell peppers and garlic. Cook the ingredients until the onions are translucent and peppers are tender, for about 15 minutes.
9. Season the spinach with sugar, cumin, turmeric, salt, and pepper.
10. Stir everything well to coat the ingredients evenly; then mix in the tomatoes, black beans, spinach, and tomato paste.
11. Heat everything for about 5 minutes, and then remove the skillet from the heat and set aside.
12. Stuff the eggplants with heaping scoops of the vegetable mixture. Sprinkle more salt and pepper to taste on top.
13. Drizzle the remaining 1 tablespoon of olive oil across the eggplants, return them to the oven, and bake until they shrivel and flatten—for 20-30 minutes.
14. Serve the eggplants, and if desired, garnish with the optional fresh thyme.
15. Enjoy right away, or, store to enjoy later!

STORAGE INFORMATION:

Storage	Temperature	Expiration date	Preparation
Airtight container M/L	Fridge at 38 – 40°F or 3°C	4-5 days after preparation	Reheat in pot or microwave
Airtight container M/L	Freezer at -1°F or -20°C	60 days after preparation	Thaw at room temperature; Reheat in pot or microwave

Note: Drizzle the eggplants with barbecue or hot sauce for a surprising kick!

Tip: Raw eggplants are very watery. Allow a part of the water to get absorbed by the paper towels before cooking.

Serves: 4 | Prep Time: ~60 min |

Nutrition Information
(per serving)
- Calories: 394 kcal
- Carbs: 39.3 g.
- Fat: 17.6 g.
- Protein: 19.7 g.
- Fiber: 3.3 g.
- Sugar: 0.7 g.

INGREDIENTS:

- 1 14-oz. package tempeh
- 3 cups vegetable broth (page 49)
- 3 cups collard greens (chopped)
- ½ cup BBQ sauce (page 184)
- 1 cup gluten-free grits
- ¼ cup white onion (diced)
- 2 tbsp. olive oil
- 2 garlic cloves (minced)
- 1 tsp. salt

Total number of ingredients: 9

METHOD:

1. Preheat the oven to 400°F / 200°C.
2. Cut the tempeh into thin slices and mix it with the BBQ sauce in a shallow baking dish. Set aside and let marinate for up to 3 hours.
3. Heat 1 tablespoon of olive oil in a frying pan over medium heat, then add the garlic and sauté until fragrant.
4. Add the collard greens and ½ teaspoon of salt and cook until the collards are wilted and dark. Remove the pan from the heat and set aside.
5. Cover the tempeh and BBQ sauce mixture with aluminum foil. Place the baking dish into the oven and bake the ingredients for 15 minutes. Uncover and continue to bake for another 10 minutes, until the tempeh is browned and crispy.
6. While the tempeh cooks, heat the remaining tablespoon of olive oil in the previously used frying pan over medium heat.
7. Cook the onions until brown and fragrant, around 10 minutes.
8. Pour in the vegetable broth and bring it to a boil; then turn the heat down to low.
9. Slowly whisk the grits into the simmering broth. Add the remaining ½ teaspoon of salt before covering the pan with a lid.
10. Let the ingredients simmer for about 8 minutes, until the grits are soft and creamy.
11. Serve the tempeh and collard greens on top of a bowl of grits and enjoy, or store for later!

STORAGE INFORMATION:

Storage	Temperature	Expiration date	Preparation
Airtight container M/L	Fridge at 38 – 40°F or 3°C	4-5 days after preparation	Reheat in pot or microwave
Airtight container M/L	Freezer at -1°F or -20°C	60 days after preparation	Thaw at room temperature; Reheat in pot or microwave

Note: For creamier grits, add a dollop of vegan butter while they cook.

Tip: Use a vegan ketchup-based barbecue sauce for the most authentic Southern flavors.

1. Stuffed Bell Peppers

Nutrition Information
(per serving)
- Calories: 171 kcal
- Carbs: 24.7 g.
- Fat: 5.2 g.
- Protein: 6.3 g.
- Fiber: 5.9 g.
- Sugar: 4.8 g.

INGREDIENTS:
- **3 cups black beans (canned or cooked)**
- **1½ cup chickpeas (canned or cooked)**
- **½ cup dry quinoa**
- **3 bell peppers (red or yellow, seeded)**
- **2 tbsp. olive oil**
- **1 sweet onion (chopped)**
- **2 tbsp. garlic (minced)**
- **2 tbsp. water**
- **1 tbsp. parsley**
- **½ cup kale (chopped, fresh or frozen)**
- **½ tbsp. dried basil**
- **Salt and pepper to taste**

Total number of ingredients: 13

METHOD:

1. When using dry beans, prepare 1 cup of dry beans and ½ cup of dry chickpeas according to the method on page 31.
2. Cook the quinoa according to the method on page 38.
3. Preheat the oven to 400°F / 200°C.
4. Slice the bell peppers in half and remove (and discard) the seeds, stem, and placenta. Place the peppers skin down on a large baking sheet and drizzle with 1 tablespoon of the olive oil, making sure the bell peppers are fully covered.
5. Bake the bell pepper halves for 10 minutes, or until the skins begin to soften.
6. While the peppers are baking, heat up 1 tablespoon of olive oil in a frying pan over medium heat.
7. Add the onion, cook until translucent (around 5 minutes), and stir in the garlic, parsley, basil, kale, and water.
8. Sauté for about 2 minutes and mix in the cooked quinoa, chickpeas, and black beans until warmed through.
9. Season the mixture to taste, stir for few minutes, and remove from heat.
10. Spoon the filling equally into the pepper halves and place them back into the oven for about 10 minutes.
11. Remove the filled bell peppers from the oven when the peppers are soft and fragrant.
12. Store for later, or, serve right away and enjoy!

STORAGE INFORMATION:

Storage	Temperature	Expiration date	Preparation
Airtight container M/L	Fridge at 38 – 40°F or 3°C	4-5 days after preparation	Reheat in pot or microwave
Airtight container M/L	Freezer at -1°F or -20°C	60 days after preparation	Thaw at room temperature; Reheat in pot or microwave

Note: Top with salsa and vegan cheese to transform this into a Tex-Mex style dinner.

Tip: Avoid over-baking the bell peppers by checking them periodically. They should be softened but not mushy.

WHOLE FOOD DINNERS

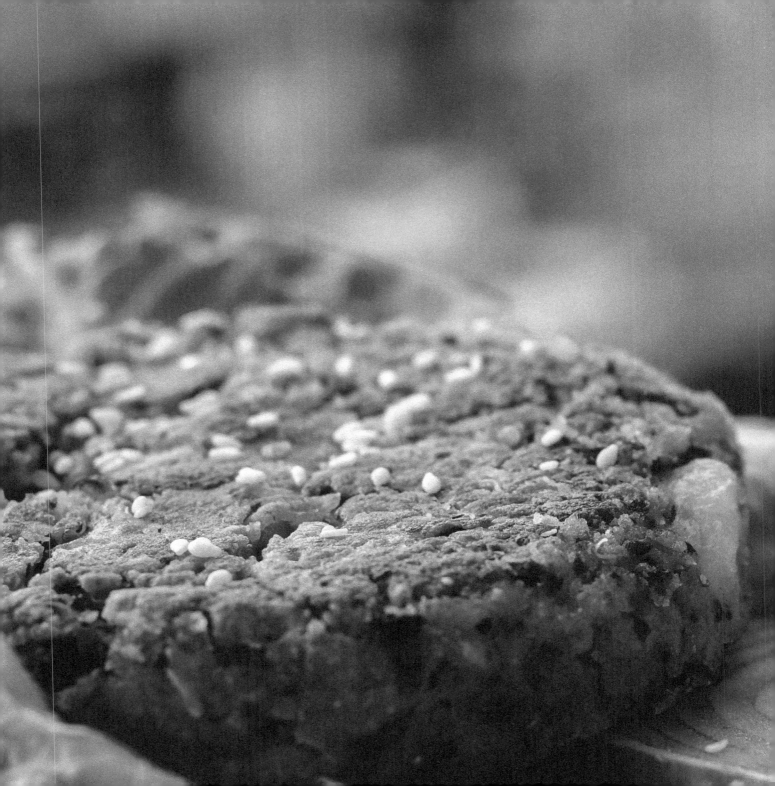

2. Black Bean & Quinoa Burgers

Serves: 3 | Prep Time: ~40 min |

Nutrition Information
(per serving)
- Calories: 200 kcal
- Carbs: 40.5 g.
- Fat: 10.6 g.
- Protein: 9.5 g.
- Fiber: 8.2 g.
- Sugar: 2.8 g.

INGREDIENTS:

- 3 cups black beans (canned or cooked)
- ½ cup dry quinoa
- ½ purple onion (chopped)
- ¼ cup bell pepper (any color, seeded and chopped)
- 2 tablespoons garlic (minced)
- ½ cup whole wheat flour
- 2 tbsp. olive oil
- ½ tsp. red pepper flakes
- ½ tsp. paprika
- 1 tsp. salt
- 1 tsp. pepper
- 4-6 large leaves of lettuce
- Optional: roasted sesame seeds

Total number of ingredients: 13

METHOD:

1. When using dry beans, prepare 1 cup of dry beans according to the method on page 31.
2. Cook the quinoa according to the method on page 38.
3. Heat 1 tablespoon of the olive oil in a frying pan over medium-high heat, and then add the onions, bell peppers, garlic, salt, and pepper.
4. Sauté until the ingredients begin to soften, for about 5 minutes. Remove the pan from the heat and let it cool down for about 10 minutes.
5. Once the veggies have cooled down, put them in a food processor along with the cooked beans, quinoa, flour, and remaining spices; pulse until it's a chunky mixture.
6. Lay out a pan covered with parchment paper and form the blended mixture into 6 evenly-sized patties.
7. Place the patties on the pan and place them in the freezer for about 5 minutes to prevent crumbling.
8. Heat the remaining oil in a frying pan over high heat and add the burgers.
9. Cook the patties until they have browned, for about 2-3 minutes per side.
10. Serve each burger wrapped in a lettuce leaf (or burger bun) and, if desired, top with the optional roasted sesame seeds. Alternatively, store to enjoy later.

Note: Add a little bit of extra water if necessary when preparing the mixture in a blender instead of a food processor.

Tip: Spray your hands with olive oil before forming the burgers to keep the mixture from sticking to them.

STORAGE INFORMATION:

Storage	Temperature	Expiration date	Preparation
Airtight container M/L	Fridge at 38 – 40°F or 3°C	3-4 days after preparation	Reheat in pot or microwave
Airtight container M/L	Freezer at -1°F or -20°C	60 days after preparation	Thaw at room temperature; Reheat in pot or microwave

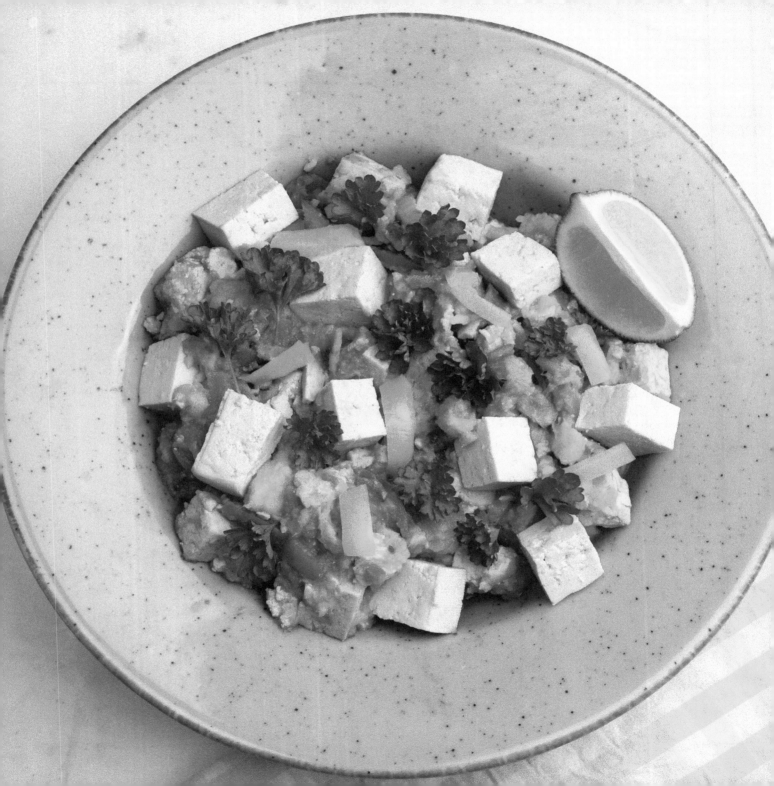

3. Sweet Potato Chili

Serves: 4 | Prep Time: ~45 min |

Nutrition Information
(per serving)
- Calories: 173 kcal
- Carbs: 15.7 g.
- Fat: 8.5 g.
- Protein: 8.6 g.
- Fiber: 5.3 g.
- Sugar: 5.6 g.

INGREDIENTS:

- 1 tbsp. extra virgin olive oil
- 1 small sweet onion (diced)
- 2 garlic cloves (minced)
- 2 medium sweet potatoes (cubed)
- 1 14-oz. block extra firm tofu (drained, cubed)
- ½ yellow bell pepper
- ½ red bell pepper
- 1 can diced tomatoes with green chilis
- ½ cup water
- 1 tbsp. chili powder
- 1 tsp. cumin
- ½ tsp. paprika
- ½ tsp. cayenne
- Salt and pepper to taste
- Optional: ¼ cup of parsley (chopped)

Total number of ingredients: 16

METHOD:

1. Heat the olive oil in a medium-sized pot over medium-high heat.
2. Sauté the garlic and onions until softened, around 5 minutes.
3. Now add the bell peppers and stir until everything is tender and fragrant, around 5 more minutes.
4. Reduce heat to low, add all remaining ingredients except the optional parsley, and stir until everything is combined thoroughly.
5. Cook the chili for 15-20 minutes, until the sweet potatoes are soft, and the liquid has thickened. Make sure to stir often and add ½ cup more water if necessary; this will result in more soup-like consistency.
6. Serve warm in a bowl, topped with the optional parsley if desired, and enjoy right away; or, store to enjoy later!

STORAGE INFORMATION:

Storage	Temperature	Expiration date	Preparation
Airtight container M/L	Fridge at 38 – 40°F or 3°C	3-4 days after preparation	Reheat in pot or microwave
Airtight container M/L	Freezer at -1°F or -20°C	60 days after preparation	Thaw at room temperature; Reheat in pot or microwave

Note: Serve with a dollop of vegan sour cream and fresh, crunchy bell peppers on top.

Tip: Peeling the potatoes is optional. Reduce prep time by not peeling.

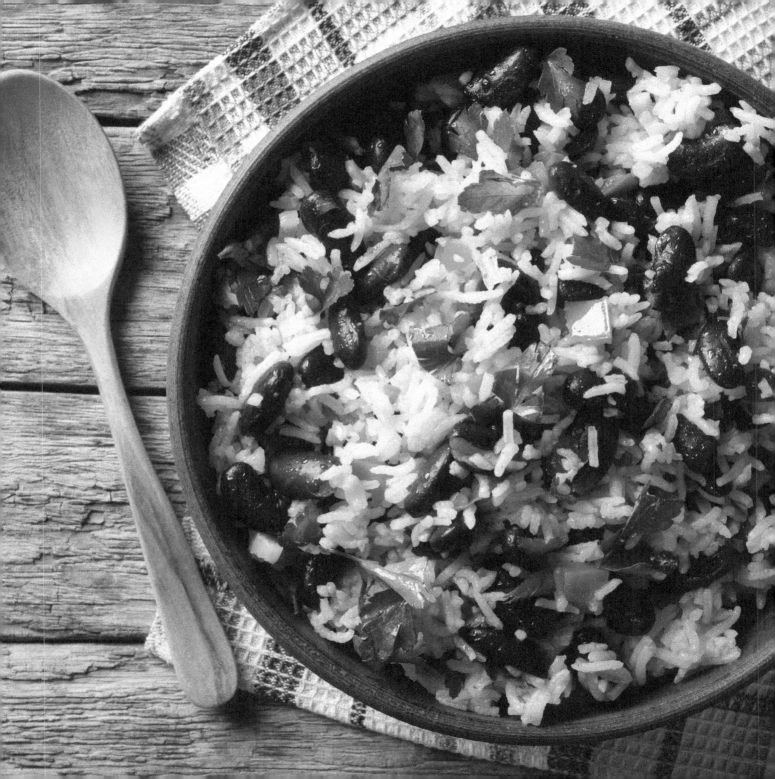

4. Red Beans & Rice

Nutrition Information
(per serving)
- Calories: 235 kcal
- Carbs: 32.3 g.
- Fat: 8.3 g.
- Protein: 7.9 g.
- Fiber: 7.3 g.
- Sugar: 2.2 g.

INGREDIENTS:
- 1 cup dry brown rice
- 4½ cups red beans (canned or cooked)
- 2 tbsp. olive oil
- ½ cup sweet onion (chopped)
- ½ cup celery ribs (diced)
- ½ cup green bell pepper (fresh or frozen, chopped)
- 1 large head of cauliflower (or 3 cups frozen cauliflower rice)
- 1 tbsp. garlic (minced)
- 2 cups of water
- 2 tsp. cumin
- 1 tsp. paprika
- 1 tsp. chili powder
- ½ tsp. basil
- ½ tsp. parsley flakes
- ½ tsp. black pepper
- Optional: ¼ cup parsley
- Optional: ¼ cup basil

Total number of ingredients: 17

METHOD:

1. Cook the brown rice according to the method on page 37.
2. When using dry beans, prepare 1½ of dry red beans according to the method on page 31.
3. Heat up the olive oil in a large frying pan over medium-high heat.
4. Add the onion, celery, and green pepper and sauté until everything has softened, in about 7 minutes.
5. Place the cauliflower into a food processor. Pulse until it resembles rice, in about a 15 seconds. (Skip this step altogether when using frozen cauliflower rice.)
6. Add the cups of water, rice, beans, and remaining ingredients to the pan.
7. Mix all the ingredients until completely distributed and cook until the cauliflower rice is soft, about 10 minutes.
8. Serve into bowls and, if desired, garnish with the optional parsley and/or basil, or, store to enjoy later!

STORAGE INFORMATION:

Storage	Temperature	Expiration date	Preparation
Airtight container M/L	Fridge at 38 – 40°F or 3°C	4-5 days after preparation	Reheat in pot or microwave
Airtight container M/L	Freezer at -1°F or -20°C	60 days after preparation	Thaw at room temperature; Reheat in pot or microwave

Note: Fresh tomatoes and jalapenos are other great garnishes for this dish.

Tip: Don't over-process the cauliflower rice. It will not hold up in the frying pan and become mushy.

5. Sweet Potato Sushi

Serves: 3 | Prep Time: ~90 min |

Nutrition Information
(per serving)
- Calories: 290 kcal
- Carbs: 39.2 g.
- Fat: 10.3 g.
- Protein: 10.3 g.
- Fiber: 6 g.
- Sugar: 11.2 g.

INGREDIENTS:

- 1 14-oz. package silken tofu (drained)
- 3-4 nori sheets
- 1 large sweet potato (peeled)
- 1 medium avocado (pitted, peeled, sliced)
- 1 cup water
- ¾ cup dry sushi rice (alternatively use brown or white rice)
- 1 tbsp. rice vinegar
- 1 tbsp. agave nectar
- 1 tbsp. coconut aminos (or tamari)

Total number of ingredients: 9

METHOD:

1. Preheat the oven to 400°F / 200°C.
2. Stir the coconut aminos (or tamari) and agave nectar together in a small bowl until it is well combined, and then set aside.
3. Cut the sweet potato into large sticks, around ½-inch thick. Place them on a baking sheet lined with parchment and coat them with the tamari/agave mixture.
4. Bake the sweet potatoes in the oven until softened—for about 25 minutes—and make sure to flip them halfway so the sides cook evenly.
5. Meanwhile, bring the sushi rice, water, and vinegar to a boil in a medium-sized pot over medium heat, and cook until liquid has evaporated, for about 10 minutes.
6. While cooking the rice, cut the block of tofu into long sticks. The sticks should look like long, thin fries. Set aside.
7. Remove the pot from heat and let the rice sit for 10-15 minutes.
8. Cover your work area with a piece of parchment paper, clean your hands, wet your fingers, and lay out a sheet of nori on the parchment paper.
9. Cover the nori sheet with a thin layer of sushi rice, while wetting the hands frequently. Leave sufficient space for rolling up the sheet.
10. Place the roasted sweet potato strips in a straight line across the width of the sheet, about an inch away from the edge closest to you.
11. Lay out the tofu and avocado slices right beside the potato sticks and use the parchment paper as an aid to roll up the nori sheet into a tight cylinder.
12. Slice the cylinder into 8 equal pieces and refrigerate. Repeat the process for the remaining nori sheets and fillings.
13. Serve chilled, or, store to enjoy this delicious sushi later!

STORAGE INFORMATION:

Storage	Temperature	Expiration date	Preparation
Airtight container M/L	Fridge at 38 – 40°F or 3°C	4-5 days after preparation	
Airtight container M/L	Freezer at -1°F or -20°C	60 days after preparation	Thaw at room temperature

Note: Serve with wasabi, ginger, and aminos for a more traditional sushi experience.

Tip: To save time and effort, use a sushi rolling mat.

6. Cuban Tempeh Buddha Bowl

Serves: 5 | Prep Time: ~15 min |

Nutrition Information
(per serving)
- Calories: 343 kcal
- Carbs: 27.4 g.
- Fat: 18.3 g.
- Protein: 17.1 g.
- Fiber: 4.7 g.
- Sugar: 0.7 g.

INGREDIENTS:

- **1 cup dry basmati rice**
- **3 cups black beans (canned or cooked)**
- **1 14-oz. package tempeh (thinly sliced)**
- **1 cup water (alternatively use vegetable broth (page 49))**
- **2 tsp. chili powder**
- **1 tsp. lime juice**
- **1¼ tsp. cumin**
- **1 pinch of salt**
- **1 tsp. turmeric**
- **2 tbsp. coconut oil**
- **1 medium avocado (pitted, peeled, diced)**

Total number of ingredients: 11

METHOD:

1. Cook the rice according the method on page 37.
2. When using dry beans, prepare 1 cup of dry black beans according the method on page 31.
3. Mix the vegetable broth, chili powder, cumin, turmeric, salt, and lime juice in a large bowl.
4. Add the tempeh and let it marinate in the fridge for up to 3 hours.
5. Heat up a frying pan with the coconut oil on medium-high heat and add the tempeh with the marinating juices.
6. Bring everything to a boil, turn down the heat, and cook over low heat until the broth is gone—10 to 15 minutes.
7. Serve the tempeh in a bowl with a scoop of rice, and top with the cooked black beans and diced avocado.

STORAGE INFORMATION:

Storage	Temperature	Expiration date	Preparation
Airtight container M/L	Fridge at 38 – 40°F or 3°C	3-4 days after preparation	Reheat in pot or microwave
Airtight container M/L	Freezer at -1°F or -20°C	60 days after preparation	Thaw at room temperature; Reheat in pot or microwave

Note: You can also top these buddha bowls with some cherry tomatoes, salsa, and/or vegan sour cream.

Tip: Undercooked tempeh will be chewy; cook the slices until they are brown and crispy for the best flavor.

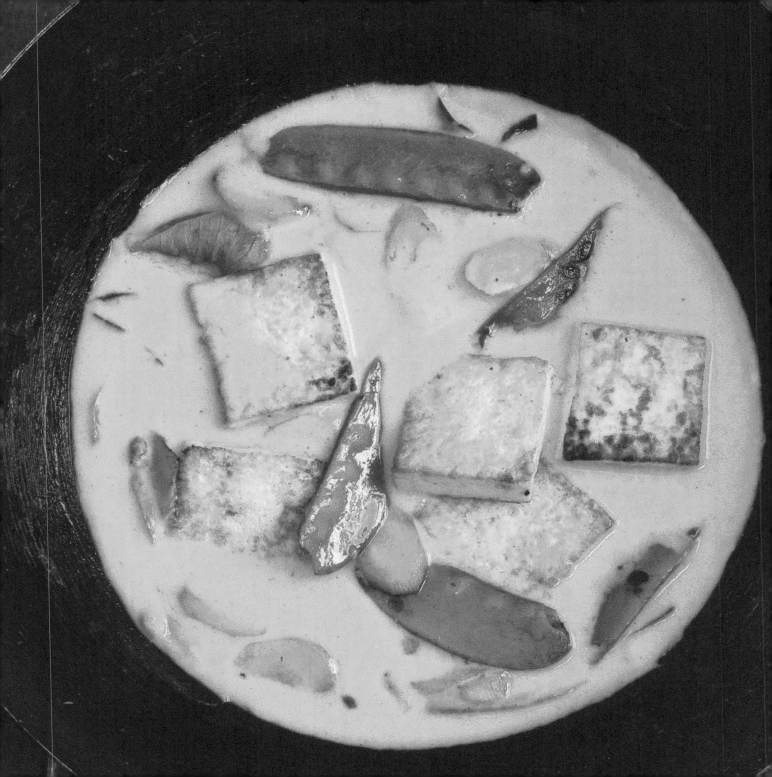

7. Coconut Tofu Curry

Serves: 2 | Prep Time: ~30 min |

Nutrition Information
(per serving)
- Calories: 449 kcal
- Carbs: 38.7 g.
- Fat: 23 g.
- Protein: 21.8 g.
- Fiber: 8.6 g.
- Sugar: 18.8 g.

INGREDIENTS:
- 1 14-oz. block firm tofu
- 2 tsp. coconut oil
- 1 medium sweet onion (diced)
- 1 13-oz. can reduced-fat coconut milk
- 1 cup fresh tomatoes (diced)
- 1 cup snap peas
- 1½ inch ginger (finely minced)
- 1 tsp. curry powder
- 1 tsp. turmeric
- 1 tsp. cumin
- ½ tsp. red pepper flakes
- 1 tsp. agave nectar (or sweet substitute)
- Salt and pepper to taste

Total number of ingredients: 14

METHOD:
1. Cut the tofu into ½-inch cubes.
2. Heat the coconut oil in a large skillet over medium-high heat.
3. Add the tofu and cook for about 5 minutes.
4. Stir in the garlic and diced onions, and sauté until the onions are transparent (for about 5 to 10 minutes); add the ginger while stirring.
5. Add in the coconut milk, tomatoes, agave nectar, snap peas, and remaining spices.
6. Combine thoroughly, cover, and cook on low heat; remove after 10 minutes of cooking.
7. For serving, scoop the curry into a bowl or over rice.
8. Enjoy right away, or, store the curry in an airtight container to enjoy later!

STORAGE INFORMATION:

Storage	Temperature	Expiration date	Preparation
Airtight container M/L	Fridge at 38 – 40°F or 3°C	4-5 days after preparation	Reheat in pot or microwave
Airtight container M/L	Freezer at -1°F or -20°C	60 days after preparation	Thaw at room temperature; Reheat in pot or microwave

Note: Add any other fresh vegetables you have on hand to this dish!

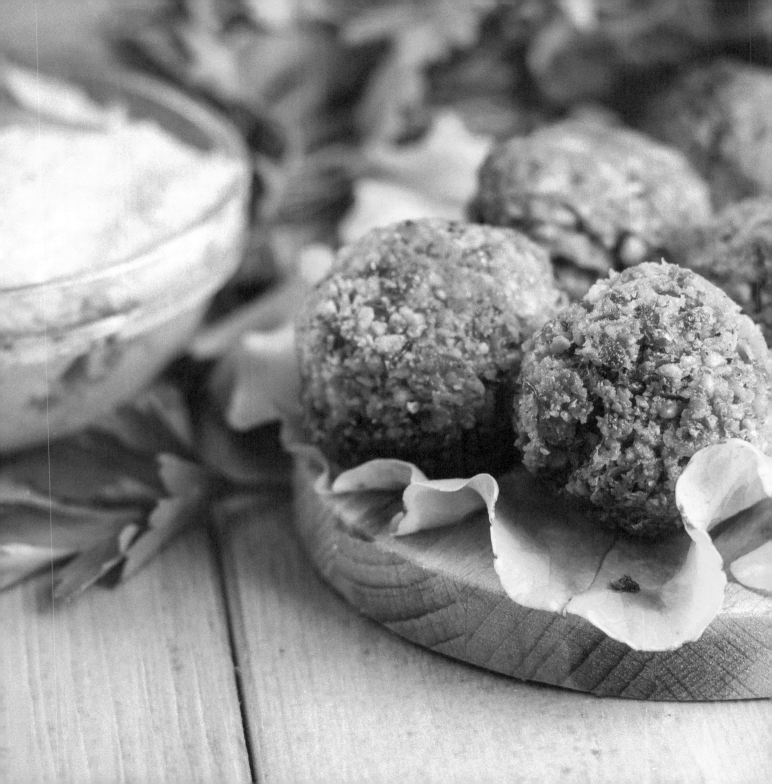

8. Tahini Falafels

Serves: 4 | Prep Time: ~30 min |

Nutrition Information
(per serving)
- Calories: 220 kcal
- Carbs: 28 g.
- Fat: 7.3 g.
- Protein: 10.5 g.
- Fiber: 8 g.
- Sugar: 3.9 g.

INGREDIENTS:

- **6 cups chickpeas (canned or cooked)**
- **1½ cup black beans (canned or cooked)**
- **2 cups broccoli florets**
- **1 garlic clove (minced)**
- **2 tsp. cumin**
- **1 tsp. olive oil**
- **½ tsp. lemon juice**
- **½ tsp. paprika**
- **¼ tsp. turmeric**
- **Dash of salt**
- **2 tbsp. tahini**

Total number of ingredients: 11

METHOD:

1. When using dry chickpeas, prepare 2 cups of dry chickpeas according to the method on page 31.
2. When using dry beans, prepare ½ cup of dry black beans according to the method on page 31.
3. Preheat the oven to 400°F / 200°C.
4. Meanwhile, place the broccoli florets in a large skillet and drizzle them with the olive oil and salt.
5. Roast the broccoli over medium-high heat until the florets are tender and brown, for 5 to 10 minutes; set aside and allow to cool a little.
6. Place the cooled broccoli with all the remaining ingredients—except the tahini—into a food processor. Blend on low for 2-3 minutes, until most large lumps are gone.
7. Line a baking pan with parchment paper. Press the falafel dough into 8 equal-sized patties and place them evenly-spaced apart on the parchment.
8. Bake the falafels until they are brown and crisp on the outside, for roughly 10 to 15 minutes. Make sure to flip them halfway through to ensure even cooking.
9. Serve with tahini as topping, or, let the falafel cool down and store for later.

STORAGE INFORMATION:

Storage	Temperature	Expiration date	Preparation
Airtight container M/L	Fridge at 38 – 40°F or 3°C	3-4 days after preparation	Reheat in pot or microwave
Airtight container M/L	Freezer at -1°F or -20°C	60 days after preparation	Thaw at room temperature; Reheat in pot or microwave

Note: These falafels also taste great in gluten-free pitas and topped with vegan garlic sauce!

Tip: The falafel will taste dry if the mixture is too chunky, and it will fall apart if blended for too long. Aim for a mixture that has some mid-sized lumps remaining.

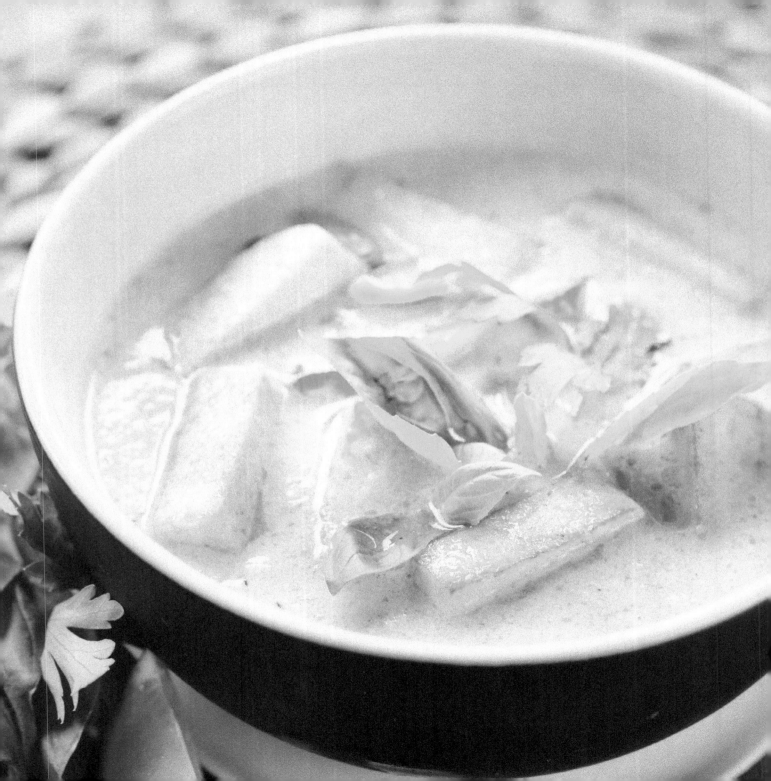

9. Green Thai Curry

Serves: 4 | Prep Time: ~30 min |

Nutrition Information
(per serving)
- Calories: 327 kcal
- Carbs: 35.6 g.
- Fat: 14.9 g.
- Protein: 12.5 g.
- Fiber: 6.8 g.
- Sugar: 10.5 g.

INGREDIENTS:
- 1 cup dry white rice
- 1 cup chickpeas (canned or cooked)
- 2 tbsp. olive oil
- 1 14-oz. package firm tofu (drained)
- 1 medium green bell pepper
- ½ white onion (diced)
- 2 tbsp. green curry paste
- 1 cup reduced-fat coconut milk
- 1 cup water (alternatively use vegetable broth (page 49))
- 1 cup peas (fresh or frozen)
- ⅓ cup fresh Thai basil (chopped)
- 2 tbsp. maple syrup (or other sweetener)
- ½ tsp. lime juice
- Dash of salt

Total number of ingredients: 14

METHOD:

1. Cook the rice according to the method on page 37.
2. Prepare ⅓ cup dry chickpeas according to the method on page 31.
3. Cut the tofu into ½-inch pieces.
4. Heat up the olive oil in a large skillet over medium-high heat and fry the tofu about 3 minutes per side.
5. Remove the skillet from the stove and set the tofu aside in a medium-sized bowl with the cooked chickpeas.
6. Using the same skillet over medium-high heat, add the bell pepper and onions and sauté until they are softened, for about 5 minutes.
7. Remove the skillet from the heat, add the green curry paste, water (or vegetable broth), and coconut milk to the skillet.
8. Stir until the curry paste is well incorporated; then add the tofu, chickpeas, and peas to the mixture and cook for 10 more minutes.
9. Drop in the Thai basil, maple syrup, and salt, and bring the mixture back up to a low cooking bubble, stirring constantly for about 3 minutes. Remove from heat.
10. Serve with rice, topped with additional chopped Thai basil, or store for later!

STORAGE INFORMATION:

Storage	Temperature	Expiration date	Preparation
2-compart-ment Airtight container M/L	Fridge at 38 – 40°F or 3°C	3-4 days after preparation	Reheat in pot or microwave
2-compart-ment Airtight container M/L	Freezer at -1°F or -20°C	60 days after preparation	Thaw at room temperature; Reheat in pot or microwave

Note: Easily customize this dish by adding more vegetables you have on hand!

Tip: Small cubes of tofu will cook too quickly for this dish. Make sure they're at least half an inch for the best results. Store the curry and rice separately.

10. Baked Enchilada Bowls

Nutrition Information
(per serving)
- Calories: 417 kcal
- Carbs: 34.6 g.
- Fat: 27.1 g.
- Protein: 15.6 g.
- Fiber: 7.2 g.
- Sugar: 6.9 g.

INGREDIENTS:

- 3 cups black beans (canned or cooked)
- 1 large sweet potato
- 4 tbsp. olive oil
- 2 cups enchilada sauce (page 186)
- 1 green bell pepper (fresh or a frozen red/green mix)
- ½ purple onion (diced)
- 1 14-oz. package firm tofu
- ½ cup cashews (chopped)
- 1 tsp. cumin
- 1 tsp. paprika
- 1 tsp. garlic powder
- 1 tsp. salt
- ½ cup vegan cheese (page 39)
- Optional: 1 tbsp. chopped jalapeños

Total number of ingredients: 14

METHOD:

1. When using dry beans, prepare 1 cup of dry black beans according to the method on page 31.
2. Preheat oven to 400°F / 200°C .
3. Cut the sweet potatoes into ¼-inch cubes and place them in a bowl with 2 tablespoons of the olive oil, the garlic powder, and ½ teaspoon of salt; toss well and make sure the sweet potatoes get coated evenly.
4. Arrange the sweet potatoes in a single layer on a baking pan. Place the pan in the oven and bake until the potato cubes begin to soften, for 15-20 minutes.
5. Meanwhile, dice up the bell pepper, onion, and tofu into ¼-inch cubes and place all in the previously used bowl with the remaining olive oil, cashews, and ½ teaspoon of salt.
6. Stir the ingredients thoroughly to make sure everything again is coated evenly.
7. After removing the potatoes from the oven, add the tofu, peppers, and onions to the baking pan and stir until combined.
8. Put the baking pan back into the oven for an additional 10 minutes, until the onions are browned, and peppers are soft.
9. Remove the pan from the oven and place the contents into a casserole dish.
10. Add the cooked black beans, enchilada sauce, and spices to the casserole dish, mixing everything until it's evenly distributed.
11. Top with a layer of vegan cheese and return to oven until it is melted, around 15 minutes.
12. Serve in a bowl topped with the optional jalapeños if desired, or store for later!

STORAGE INFORMATION:

Storage	Temperature	Expiration date	Preparation
Airtight container M/L	Fridge at 38 – 40°F or 3°C	4-5 days after preparation	Reheat in pot or microwave
Airtight container M/L	Freezer at -1°F or -20°C	60 days after preparation	Thaw at room temperature; Reheat in pot or microwave

Note: Raw purple onions, avocado slices, and/or salsa make great toppings.

Tip: Don't overcook the sweet potatoes! They'll continue cooking later in the recipe.

1. Gluten-Free Energy Crackers

Nutrition Information
(per serving)
- Calories: 209 kcal
- Carbs: 10.3 g.
- Fat: 15.6 g.
- Protein: 6.9 g.
- Fiber: 6.3 g.
- Sugar: 0.7 g.

INGREDIENTS:

- ¼ cup flax seeds
- ¼ cup chia seeds
- ¾ cup water
- 1 tbsp. garlic (minced)
- ½ tbsp. dried onion flakes
  (alternatively use onion
  powder)
- ½ cup pumpkin seeds
  (chopped)
- ¼ cup peanuts (crushed)
- ¼ cup cashews (crushed)
- ¼ cup sesame seeds
- ¼ tsp. paprika powder
- Salt and pepper to taste

Total number of ingredients: 12

METHOD:

1. Preheat the oven to 350°F / 175°C.
2. Take a large bowl and combine the water, garlic, onion flakes, and paprika. Whisk until everything is combined thoroughly.
3. To the same bowl, add the flax seeds, chia seeds, pumpkin seeds, peanuts, cashews, and sesame seeds.
4. Stir everything well, while adding pinches of salt and pepper to taste, until it is thoroughly combined.
5. Line a baking sheet with parchment paper and spread out the mixture in a thin and even layer across the parchment paper.
6. Bake for 20-25 minutes.
7. Remove the pan from the oven and flip over the flat chunk so that the other side can crisp.
8. Cut the chunk into squares or triangles, depending on preference and put the pan back into the oven and bake until the bars have turned golden brown, around 30 minutes.
9. Allow the crackers to cool before serving or storing. Enjoy!

Note: Experiment with extra seeds, nuts, and spices. Try different combinations for an endless variety of energy cracker flavors!

Tip: A thin layer of the mixture will make thin crackers, while a thicker layer will make thicker crackers. Thicker crackers will take longer to crisp in the oven.

STORAGE INFORMATION:

Storage	Temperature	Expiration date	Preparation
Airtight container L	Fridge at 38 – 40°F or 3°C	4-5 days after preparation	Reheat in pot or microwave
Airtight container L	Freezer at -1°F or -20°C	60 days after preparation	Thaw at room temperature

QUICK ENERGY & RECOVERY SNACKS

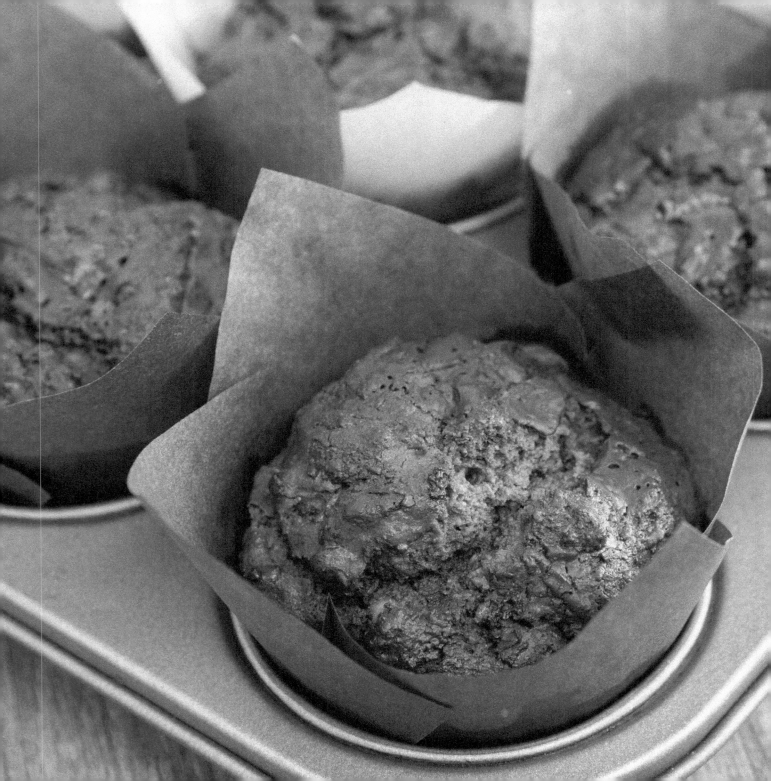

2. Chocolate, Quinoa & Zucchini Muffins

Serves: 8 | Prep Time: ~40 min |

Nutrition Information
(per serving)
- Calories: 354 kcal
- Carbs: 30.4 g.
- Fat: 19.4 g.
- Protein: 14.2 g.
- Fiber: 3.7 g.
- Sugar: 19.7 g.

INGREDIENTS:
- ½ cup dry quinoa
- 2 tbsp. coconut oil
- 1½ cup almond flour
- ½ cup walnuts (chopped)
- 2 large bananas
- ½ cup applesauce
- ¼ cup maple syrup
- ½ cup zucchini (shredded)
- 1 cup vegan protein powder (vanilla or chocolate flavor)
- ½ cup vegan dark chocolate chips (alternatively use cacao powder)
- 3-5 tbsp. almond milk
- 2 tsp. baking powder
- ½ tsp. cinnamon
- ½ tsp. vanilla extract
- ½ tsp. nutmeg
- pinch of salt
- Optional: ½ cup water

Total number of ingredients: 17

METHOD:

1. Cook the quinoa according to the method on page 38 and set aside.
2. Preheat the oven to 400°F / 200°C .
3. Line an 8-cup muffin pan with baking cups, spray with coconut oil, and set aside.
4. In a large bowl, mix together the flour, cooked quinoa, nutmeg, walnuts, cinnamon, salt, and baking powder.
5. Take a second bowl and mash the bananas with a fork, and then combine the mashed bananas with the applesauce.
6. Stir in the vanilla, maple syrup, protein powder, and almond milk until all the ingredients are distributed evenly; if necessary, add the optional water.
7. Combine the separate mixtures into one large bowl. Stir until the batter is smooth and lumps have dissolved.
8. Finally, carefully fold in the shredded zucchini and chocolate chips.
9. Fill each of the muffin cups halfway.
10. Bake in the oven until the muffins are fluffy all the way through, for about 20 minutes.
11. Remove from the oven and cool for at least 15 minutes before serving or storing and enjoy!

STORAGE INFORMATION:

Storage	Temperature	Expiration date	Preparation
Airtight container M/L	Fridge at 38 – 40°F or 3°C	5-6 days after preparation	Reheat in pot or microwave
Airtight container M/L	Freezer at -1°F or -20°C	60 days after preparation	Thaw at room temperature; Reheat in pot or microwave

Note: Add extra chocolate chips or oatmeal flakes on top of the batter before baking for even tastier muffins, that are nutritious too!

Tip: If your batter seems too runny, consider adding less almond flour or water. If your dough is too dry, add more almond milk or water.

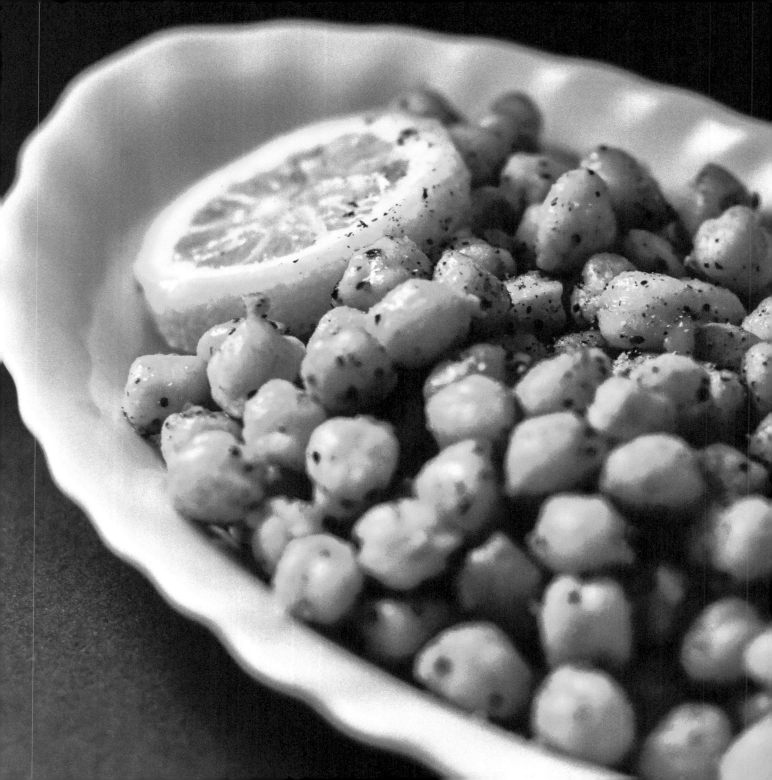

3. Spicy Chickpea Poppers

Serves: 3 | Prep Time: ~45 min |

Nutrition Information
(per serving)
- Calories: 192 kcal
- Carbs: 21.5 g.
- Fat: 7.8 g.
- Protein: 9.1 g.
- Fiber: 12.8 g.
- Sugar: 1.4 g.

INGREDIENTS:
- **6 cups chickpeas (canned or cooked)**
- **1 tbsp. coconut oil**
- **½ tsp. salt**
- **½ tsp. chili powder**
- **½ tsp. garlic powder**
- **¼ tsp. onion powder**
- **¼ tsp. cumin**
- **¼ tsp. paprika**
- **¼ tsp. cayenne**

Total number of ingredients: 9

METHOD:
1. When using dry chickpeas, prepare 2 cups of dry chickpeas according to the method on page 31.
2. Preheat the oven 400°F / 200°C.
3. Line a baking sheet with parchment paper and set aside.
4. Put the chickpeas on a large plate and pat them dry.
5. Place on the baking sheet and coat with coconut oil, salt, onion powder, and garlic powder.
6. Bake the chickpeas in the oven until they are brown and fragrant—around 25-30 minutes—while stirring every 5-10 minutes to prevent burning.
7. Take the chickpeas out of the oven and let them cool for about 5 minutes.
8. Put the chickpeas into a bowl and mix in the remaining spices until evenly coated.
9. Add salt to taste and serve warm.

STORAGE INFORMATION:

Storage	Temperature	Expiration date	Preparation
Airtight container S/M/L	Fridge at 38 – 40°F or 3°C	5 days after preparation	Reheat in the oven or a skillet
Freezer not recommended			

Note: Feel free to substitute olive oil for the coconut oil for a more savory flavor.

Tip: You'll hear the chickpeas pop as they cook; this means they are heating properly.

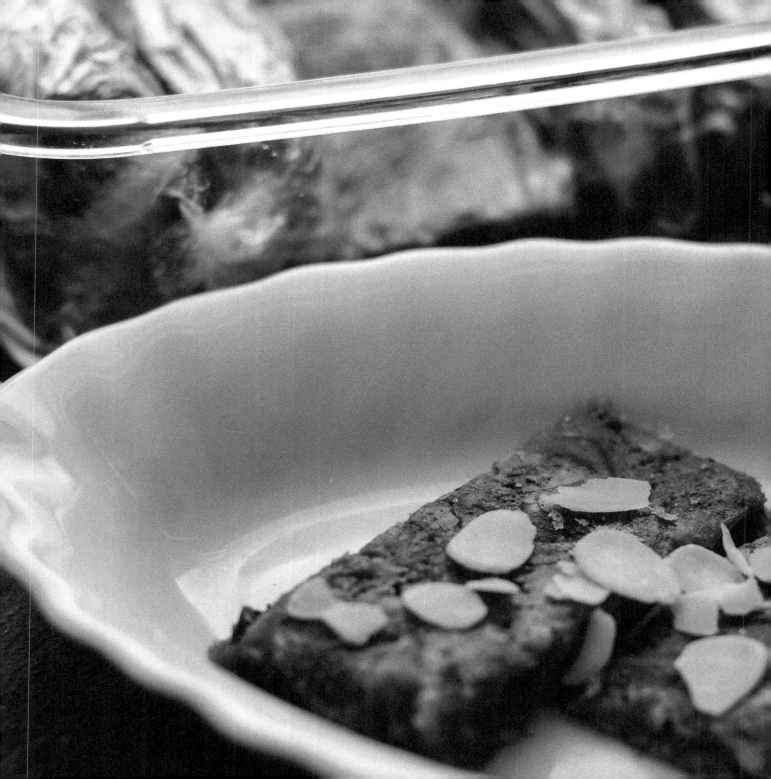

4. Almond & Date Protein Bars

Nutrition Information
(per serving)
- Calories: 261 kcal
- Carbs: 15.6 g.
- Fat: 17.4 g.
- Protein: 10.5 g.
- Fiber: 2.9 g.
- Sugar: 8.2 g.

INGREDIENTS:

- **1 cup natural almond butter**
- **½ cup vegan chocolate protein powder**
- **½ cup pitted dates**
- **¼ cup dried cranberries**
- **¼ cup chopped almonds**
- **¼ cup flax seeds**
- **2 tbsp. applesauce (page 189)**
- **1 tsp. coconut oil**

Total number of ingredients: 8

METHOD:

1. Line an 8x8" baking dish with parchment paper and set aside.
2. Add all the ingredients into a food processor and blend until it forms a tacky, thick dough.
3. Press the dough into the baking dish, while making sure to properly press it into each corner; use your hands to pack the batter down evenly across the entire pan.
4. Place in the refrigerator for around 2 hours to cool, or 1 hour in the freezer.
5. Cut into 8 equal-sized bars and store, or, enjoy the bars right away.

STORAGE INFORMATION:

Storage	Temperature	Expiration date	Preparation
Airtight container S/M/L or Ziploc bag	Fridge at 38 – 40°F or 3°C	7 days after preparation	Serve chilled
Airtight container or Ziploc bag	Freezer at -1°F or -20°C	60 days after preparation	Thaw at room temperature

Note: Sprinkle carob chips on top of the batter before baking for a sweeter, chocolatey treat!

Tip: If the batter is too wet, add more protein powder until it thickens. If it's too dry, add more coconut oil.

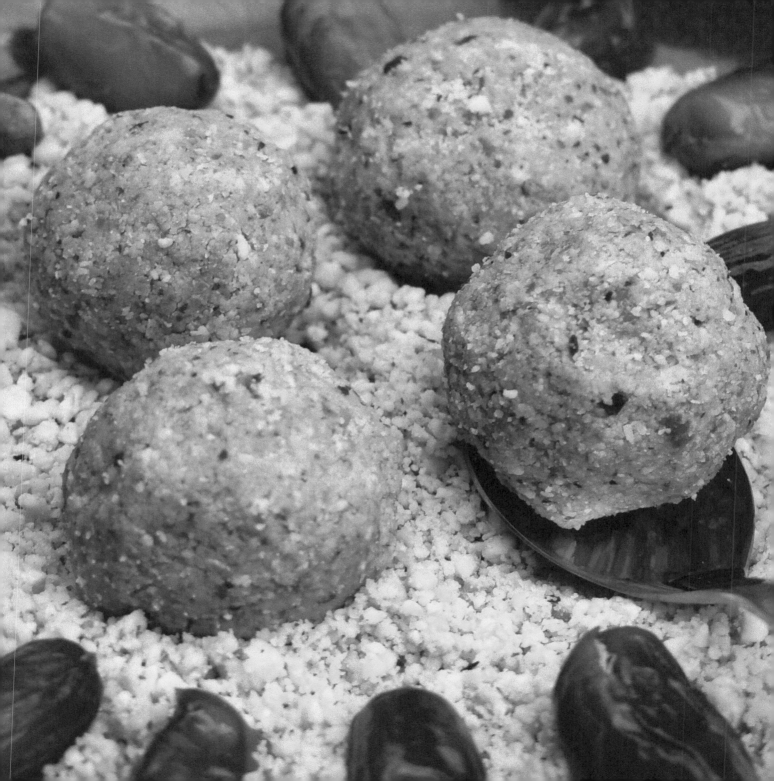

5. Matcha Energy Balls

Nutrition Information
(per serving)
- Calories: 335 kcal
- Carbs: 21.3 g.
- Fat: 21.25 g.
- Protein: 14.6 g.
- Fiber: 4.7 g.
- Sugar: 12.8 g.

INGREDIENTS:
- **1 cup raw cashews**
- **½ cup pistachios**
- **½ cup pitted dates, packed**
- **½ cup vanilla vegan protein powder**
- **¼ cup finely shredded coconut**
- **¼ cup crushed hazelnuts**
- **1 tbsp. matcha powder**
- **1 tbsp. maple syrup**

Total number of ingredients: 8

METHOD:

1. Add all the ingredients—except the hazelnuts—to a food processor and blend on low until everything is finely crushed and combined, around 45 seconds.
2. Use a tablespoon to scoop out rounded heaps of the mixture, and then use your hands to roll them into balls.
3. Pour the crushed hazelnuts out into a bowl and roll the matcha balls in the hazelnuts until they are evenly coated on all sides.
4. Refrigerate for about 30 minutes until the balls are solid, and store or serve right away!

STORAGE INFORMATION:

Storage	Temperature	Expiration date	Preparation
Airtight container S/M/L or Ziploc bag	Fridge at 38 – 40°F or 3°C	5 days after preparation	Serve chilled or thaw to room temperature
Airtight container or Ziploc bag	Freezer at -1°F or -20°C	60 days after preparation	Thaw at room temperature

Note: You can also roll the matcha balls in crushed pistachios or shredded coconut.

Tip: Press the matcha balls into the crushed hazelnuts to ensure they don't fall off once the dough hardens.

6. Raw Lemon Pie Bars

Serves: 6 | Prep Time: ~10 min |

Nutrition Information
(per serving)
- Calories: 272 kcal
- Carbs: 34.9 g.
- Fat: 10.7 g.
- Protein: 8.9 g.
- Fiber: 6.5 g.
- Sugar: 24.7 g.

INGREDIENTS:

- ¼ cup chia seeds
- ¼ cup pecan pieces
- ⅓ cup raw cashews
- ⅓ cup sunflower seeds
- 2 cups of pitted dates
- ½ cup vegan protein powder
  (vanilla flavor)
- 2 tbsp. organic lemon juice
  (or lime juice)
- ¼ tsp. salt

Total number of ingredients: 8

METHOD:

1. Soak the chia seeds according to the method on page 31 and drain the excess water.
2. Place the pecans, cashews, chia seeds, and sunflower seeds in a food processor and pulse on low until it is a crumbly mixture.
3. Add the dates, lemon or lime juice, and salt to the processor. Continue pulsing while adding protein powder until the mixture is a bit chunky but doughy.
4. Transfer the dough to a baking sheet lined with parchment paper and press it out with your fingers or rolling pin until it forms a ½-inch thick square.
5. Place the sheet pan into the freezer until the chunk is solid, or for about 1 hour.
6. Slice the chunk into 8 equally-sized bars. Store, or enjoy right away.

STORAGE INFORMATION:

Storage	Temperature	Expiration date	Preparation
Airtight container S/M/L or Ziploc bag	Fridge at 38 – 40°F or 3°C	5 days after preparation	Reheat in pot or microwave
Airtight container or Ziploc bag	Freezer at -1°F or -20°C	60 days after preparation	Thaw at room temperature; Reheat in pot or microwave

Note: Substituting hazelnuts for cashews will add a yummy twist to these citrus-y bars!

Tip: Pack down the dates for the best results.

7. High Protein Black Bean Dip

Nutrition Information
(per serving)
- Calories: 398 kcal
- Carbs: 63 g.
- Fat: 6.6 g.
- Protein: 21.3 g.
- Fiber: 16 g.
- Sugar: 3.5 g.

INGREDIENTS:

- **4 cups black beans
  (cooked, rinsed, drained)**
- **2 tbsp. minced garlic**
- **2 tbsp. Italian seasoning**
- **2 tbsp. onion powder**
- **1 tbsp. olive oil**
- **1 tbsp. lemon juice**
- **¼ tsp. salt + salt to taste**

Total number of ingredients: 7

METHOD:

1. Place black beans in a large bowl and mash them with a fork until everything is mostly smooth.
2. Stir in the remaining ingredients and incorporate thoroughly. The mixture should be smooth and creamy.
3. Add some additional salt and lemon juice to taste and serve at room temperature.

STORAGE INFORMATION:

Storage	Temperature	Expiration date	Preparation
Airtight container S/M/L	Fridge at 38 – 40°F or 3°C	5 days after preparation	Reheat in microwave or serve cold
Airtight container S/M/L	Freezer at -1°F or -20°C	30 days after preparation	Reheat in microwave or serve cold

Note: Serve with slices of broccoli, carrots, and celery for a classic veggie dip.

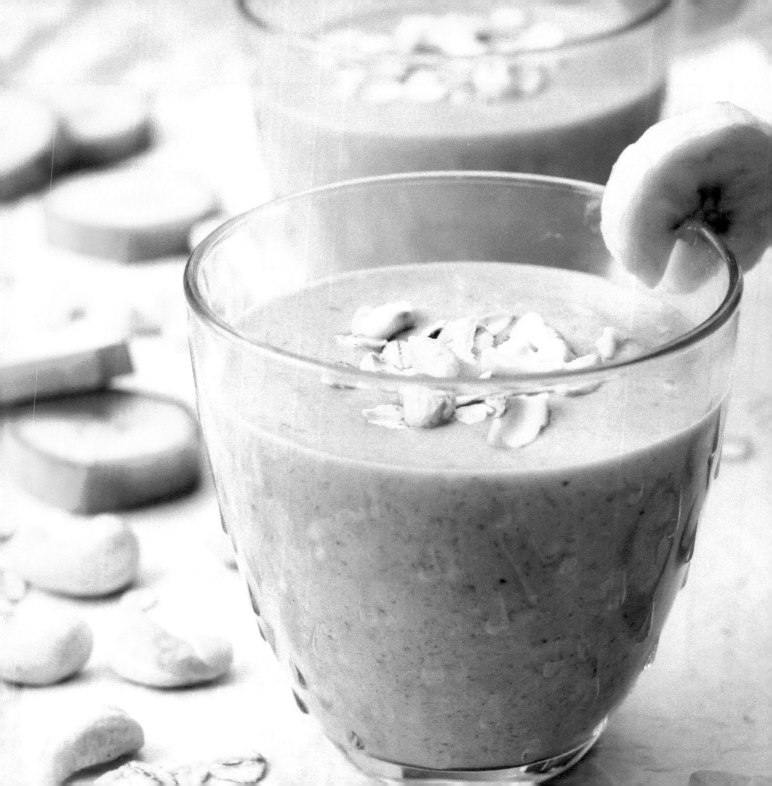

8. High Protein Cake Batter Smoothie

Nutrition Information
(per serving)
- Calories: 241 kcal
- Carbs: 27.2 g.
- Fat: 7.6 g.
- Protein: 16 g.
- Fiber: 2.5 g.
- Sugar: 12.4 g.

INGREDIENTS:
- 1 large banana (frozen)
- 1 cup almond milk
  (alternatively use soymilk)
- ¼ cup quick oats
- 4 tbsp. vegan protein powder
  (chocolate flavor)
- 1 tbsp. cashew butter
- 1 tsp. cinnamon
- 1 tsp. pure vanilla extract
- ¼ tsp. nutmeg

Total number of ingredients: 8

METHOD:
1. Mix the oats and almond milk in a small bowl or jar.
2. Place the bowl in the fridge until the oats have softened, for about 1 hour.
3. Add the oats and milk mixture along with the remaining ingredients to a blender.
4. Blend on high speed until it is smooth, and all lumps have disappeared.
5. Serve in tall glasses with an extra sprinkle of cinnamon on top, or store to enjoy later.

STORAGE INFORMATION:

Storage	Temperature	Expiration date	Preparation
Airtight thermos, cup, or jar	Fridge at 38 – 40°F or 3°C	2-3 days after preparation	Serve chilled
Airtight container S/M or jar	Freezer at -1°F or -20°C	60 days after preparation	Thaw in the fridge

Note: Other butters, like almond or peanut butter, will also work in this smoothie.

Tip: Soaking the oats prevents them from becoming gritty after blending.

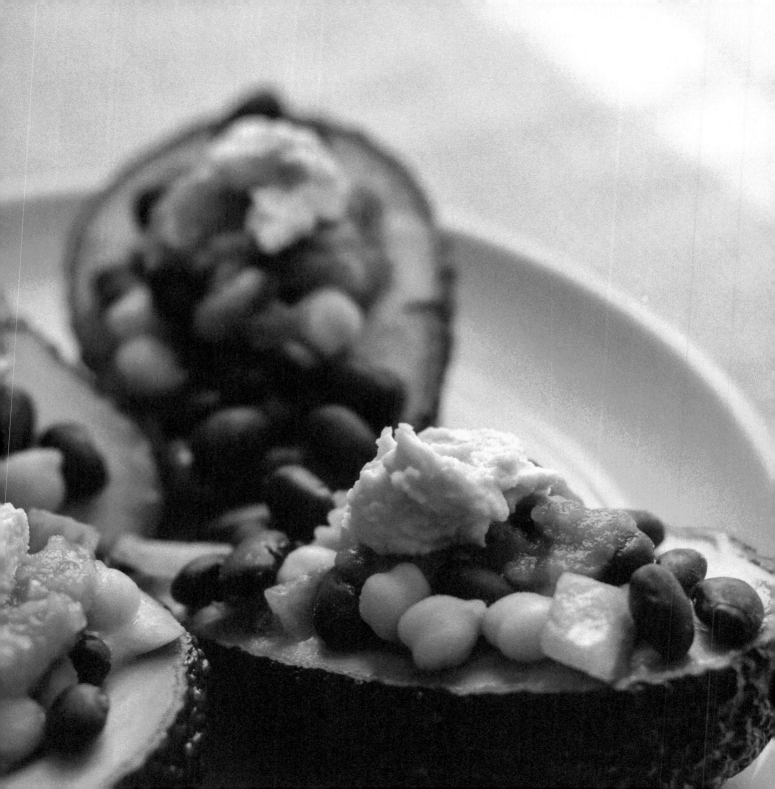

9. Southwest Stuffed Avocado Bowls

Serves: 4 | Prep Time: ~30 min |

Nutrition Information
(per serving)
- Calories: 351 kcal
- Carbs: 32.6 g.
- Fat: 20 g.
- Protein: 10 g.
- Fiber: 15.6 g.
- Sugar: 7 g.

INGREDIENTS:

- 3 cups black beans (canned or cooked)
- ¾ cup chickpeas (canned or cooked)
- 1 cup water or vegetable broth (page 49)
- ½ purple onion (chopped)
- 1 tsp. garlic powder
- ½ tsp. chili powder
- ½ tsp. cumin
- ¼ tsp. paprika
- 4 small-to-medium avocados (halved)
- 1 tsp. lime juice
- 1 pinch of salt
- ¼ cup salsa (page 187)
- ¼ cup hummus (page 56)

Total number of ingredients: 13

METHOD:

1. When using dry beans, prepare 1 cup of dry black beans according to the method on page 31.
2. When using dry chickpeas, prepare ¼ cup of chickpeas according to the method on page 31.
3. Heat the water or vegetable broth in a medium-sized pot over medium-high heat.
4. Add the cooked black beans, chickpeas, onions, and all the spices.
5. Stir well to combine all the ingredients and softly cook the mixture until the water has almost evaporated, for about 10 to 15 minutes.
6. Meanwhile, sprinkle the avocado halves with the lime juice and some salt.
7. Store the ingredients separately, or, serve the avocado halves with a scoop of the beans mixture and top with some hummus and salsa.

STORAGE INFORMATION:

Storage	Temperature	Expiration date	Preparation
3-compartment airtight container M/L	Fridge at 38 – 40°F or 3°C	1-2 days after preparation	
3-compartment airtight container M/L	Freezer at -1°F or -20°C	60 days after preparation	Thaw at room temperature

Note: Use a 3-compartment container or separate containers to store the bean mixture, hummus, and salsa. Avocado halves are best cut fresh before serving.

Tip: When storing avocado halves in the fridge, squeeze lime juice over them before placing in the refrigerator to prevent browning.

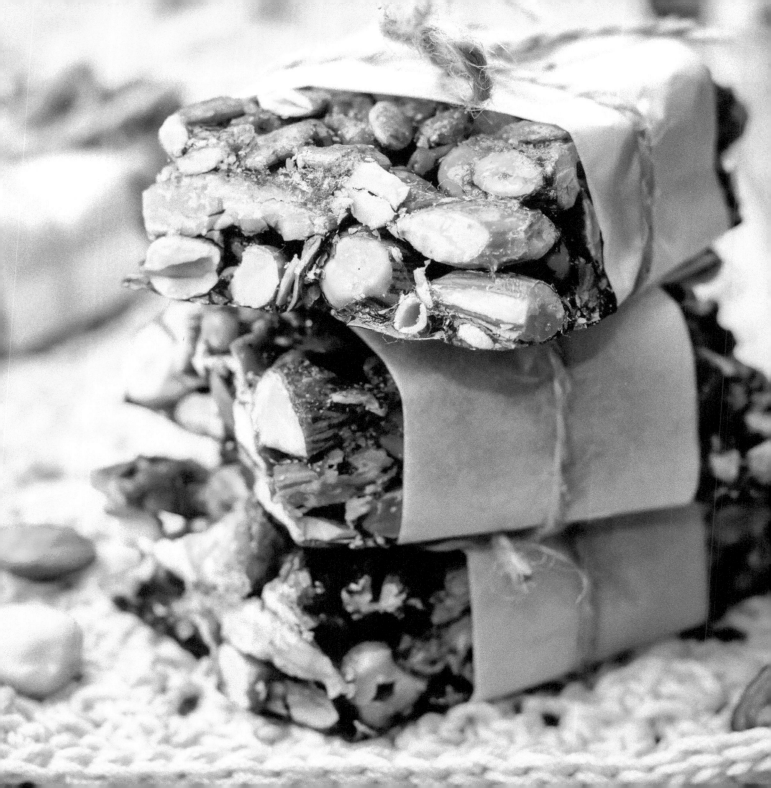

10. Candied Protein Trail Mix Bars

Serves: 8 | Prep Time: ~20 min |

Nutrition Information
(per serving)
- Calories: 387 kcal
- Carbs: 19.5 g.
- Fat: 28 g.
- Protein: 14 g.
- Fiber: 7.4 g.
- Sugar: 8 g.

INGREDIENTS:

- **2 cups raw almonds**
- **2 cups raw pecan halves**
- **1 cup raw walnuts**
- **¼ cup maple syrup**
- **½ cup vegan protein powder (vanilla or chocolate flavor)**
- **¼ tsp. cinnamon**
- **¼ tsp. salt**

Total number of ingredients: 7

METHOD:

1. Heat a large non-stick frying pan over medium-low heat, and then add the nuts, maple syrup, and protein powder. Stir constantly until the ingredients become thick and tacky, around 8-10 minutes.
2. Sprinkle the salt and cinnamon over the nut mixture and heat for 2 additional minutes before removing the skillet from the heat.
3. Line a shallow pan with parchment paper. Spread out the mixture and allow it to cool down completely.
4. To serve, separate the chunk into 8 pieces and enjoy, or, store for later!

STORAGE INFORMATION:

Storage	Temperature	Expiration date	Preparation
Airtight container L or Ziploc bag	Fridge at 38 – 40°F or 3°C	30 days after preparation	Eat at room temperature.

Note: Nutmeg, cardamom, and pumpkin spice are other great additions to this trail mix.

Tip: The syrup will harden as it cools. Apply the runny mixture to the pan lined with parchment paper when it's still warm.

11. No-Bake Almond-Rice Treats

Serves: 8 | Prep Time: ~20 min |

Nutrition Information
(per serving)
- Calories: 191 kcal
- Carbs: 13.2 g.
- Fat: 11.2 g.
- Protein: 9.3 g.
- Fiber: 1.2 g.
- Sugar: 6.4 g.

INGREDIENTS:

- ¼ cup brown rice syrup
- 2 tbsp. almond milk
- ¾ cup vegan protein powder
  (chocolate or flavor of choice)
- ¾ cup almond butter
- 4 cups puffy rice cereal
- 1 tbsp. pure vanilla extract
- ⅓ cup almonds (crushed)
- ⅓ cup shredded coconut
- Optional: ⅓ cup hazelnuts
  (crushed)
- ¼ tsp. salt

Total number of ingredients: 10

METHOD:

1. Line an 8x8" square baking dish with parchment paper and set it aside.
2. Take a large saucepan and put it over low heat.
3. Heat the brown rice syrup, almond milk, protein powder, almond butter, and salt in this pan until bubbly.
4. Continue to lower the heat and stir in the vanilla extract and rice cereal. Mix all the ingredients until evenly coated.
5. Transfer the warm mixture to the baking dish lined with parchment paper. Spread the mixture out using your fingers or a spoon until it's an even thickness all the way across the dish.
6. Sprinkle the top of the mixture with the crushed almonds, shredded coconut, and optional crushed hazelnuts.
7. Place in the freezer until the chunk is firm, for about 1 hour.
8. Remove and slice the chunk into 8 even bars.
9. Store for later or enjoy right away!

Note: Chopped peanuts, cashews, or walnuts also taste great in or on top of these protein bars!

Tip: Drizzle the bars with some melted vegan chocolate for an elevated presentation. Do so before putting the chunk in the freezer or after cutting the bars.

STORAGE INFORMATION:

Storage	Temperature	Expiration date	Preparation
Airtight container L or Ziploc bag	Fridge at 38 – 40°F or 3°C	6-7 days after preparation	Serve chilled
Airtight container L or Ziploc bag	Freezer at -1°F or -20°C	60 days after preparation	Thaw in the fridge

12. Sunflower Protein Bars

Nutrition Information
(per serving)
- Calories: 188 kcal
- Carbs: 21.9 g.
- Fat: 6.8 g.
- Protein: 9.6 g.
- Fiber: 1.3 g.
- Sugar: 9.4 g.

INGREDIENTS:
- **1 cup old fashioned oats**
- **1 cup puffy rice cereal**
- **1 cup vegan protein powder (chocolate flavor)**
- **½ cup maple syrup**
- **½ cup sunflower butter**
- **2 tsp. pure vanilla extract**
- **1 tsp. cinnamon**
- **¼ tsp. nutmeg**
- **¼ tsp. salt**

Total number of ingredients: 9

METHOD:
1. In a large bowl, mix together the oats, rice cereal, protein powder, cinnamon, nutmeg, and salt; set aside.
2. Take a smaller bowl, add the sunflower butter, maple syrup, and heat in the microwave for 30 seconds.
3. Remove the melted sunflower butter mixture from the microwave and mix the heated ingredients into the large bowl with the dry ingredients.
4. Stir everything thoroughly, add the vanilla extract, and use a whisk to mix everything together until all the lumps have dissolved to create a smooth mixture.
5. Spread the mixture into a shallow dish lined with parchment paper, and then pack it down firmly with a spoon to make sure no air bubbles remain.
6. Transfer the dish to the freezer and let it sit for at least 20 minutes.
7. Take the dish out and cut the chunk into 6 equal-sized bars; store or enjoy right away!

STORAGE INFORMATION:

Storage	Temperature	Expiration date	Preparation
Airtight container M	Fridge at 38 – 40°F or 3°C	4-5 days after preparation	
Airtight container M	Freezer at -1°F or -20°C	60 days after preparation	Thaw at room temperature

Note: Top these bars with crushed seeds, nuts, or rasped coconut!

Tip: Add brown rice syrup to the ingredients for stickier rice treats.

13. Mocha Chocolate Brownie Bars

Serves: 3 | Prep Time: ~15 min |

Nutrition Information
(per serving)
- Calories: 213 kcal
- Carbs: 17.3 g.
- Fat: 3.8 g.
- Protein: 27.3 g.
- Fiber: 3.7 g.
- Sugar: 6.1 g.

INGREDIENTS:
- **2½ cups vegan protein powder (chocolate or vanilla)**
- **½ cup cocoa powder**
- **½ cup old-fashioned or quick oats**
- **1 tsp. pure vanilla extract**
- **¼ tsp. nutmeg**
- **2 tbsp. agave nectar**
- **1 cup brewed coffee (cold)**

Total number of ingredients: 7

METHOD:
1. Line a square baking dish with parchment paper and set it aside.
2. Mix the dry ingredients together in a large bowl.
3. Slowly incorporate the agave nectar, vanilla extract, and cold coffee while stirring constantly until all the lumps in the mixture have disappeared.
4. Pour the batter into the dish, while making sure to press it into the corners.
5. Place the dish into the refrigerator until firm, or for about 4 hours. Alternatively use the freezer for just 1 hour.
6. Slice the chunk into 6 even squares, and enjoy, share, or store!

STORAGE INFORMATION:

Storage	Temperature	Expiration date	Preparation
Airtight container M/L or Ziploc bag	Fridge at 38 – 40°F or 3°C	4-5 days after preparation	Serve chilled
Airtight container M/L or Ziploc bag	Freezer at -1°F or -20°C	60 days after preparation	Thaw at room temperature

Note: These brownies are even better when they're garnished with crushed hazelnuts or almonds!

Tip: Press the batter down firmly in the dish with a spoon to remove any air bubbles.

14. Cranberry Vanilla Protein Bars

Serves: 4 | Prep Time: ~15 min |

Nutrition Information
(per serving)
- Calories: 243 kcal
- Carbs: 22.9 g.
- Fat: 9.6 g.
- Protein: 16.1 g.
- Fiber: 3.1 g.
- Sugar: 9.9 g.

INGREDIENTS:

- **1 cup old-fashioned oats**
- **2 cups vegan protein powder (vanilla flavor)**
- **⅓ cup shredded coconut**
- **½ cup cashew butter**
- **½ cup dried cranberries**
- **¼ cup maple syrup**
- **¼ cup chia seeds**
- **1 tbsp. almond or soymilk**
- **1 tbsp. pure vanilla extract**

Total number of ingredients: 9

METHOD:

1. Line a square 8x8" baking dish with parchment paper and set it aside.
2. Add the oats, protein powder, and shredded coconut to a food processor and blend until they resemble a fine powder.
3. Transfer the blended ingredients to a large mixing bowl and add the remaining ingredients; mix with a spoon until everything is thoroughly combined.
4. Move the dough to the baking dish and press it down evenly until flattened as much as possible.
5. Place the dish into the freezer until set and firm, around 1½ hours.
6. To serve, slice the chunk into 8 even bars, and enjoy, share, or store!

STORAGE INFORMATION:

Storage	Temperature	Expiration date	Preparation
Airtight container M/L or Ziploc bag	Fridge at 38 – 40°F or 3°C	6-7 days after preparation	Serve chilled or at room temperature
Airtight container M/L or Ziploc bag	Freezer at -1°F or -20°C	60 days after preparation	Thaw at room temperature

Note: Dried cherries also make a great addition to these bars!

Tip: Use another flavor plant-based protein powder to alter the taste of these bars.

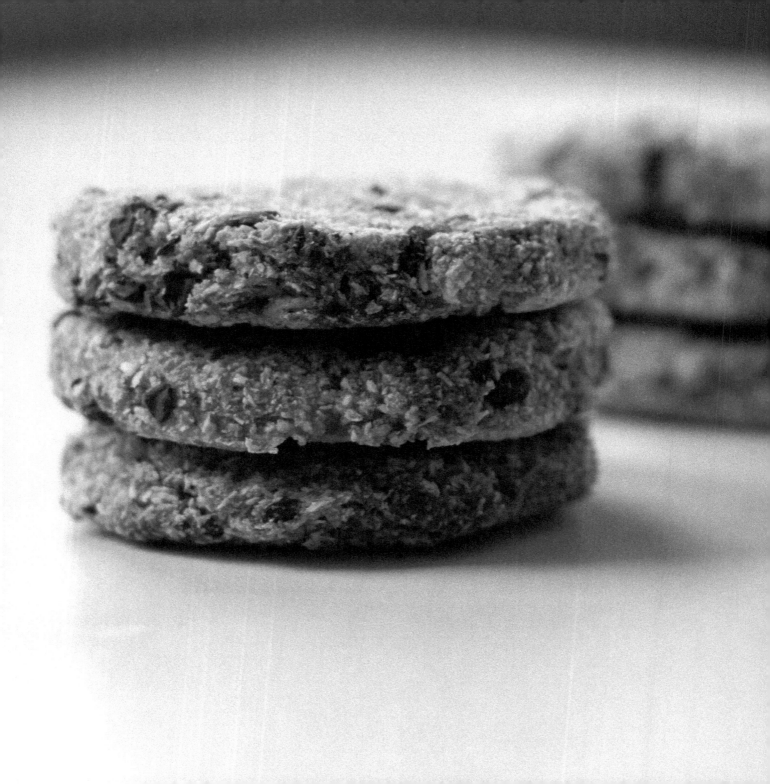

15. Peanut Butter & Banana Cookies

Serves: 8 | Prep Time: ~20 min |

Nutrition Information
(per serving)
- Calories: 220 kcal
- Carbs: 20.2 g.
- Fat: 11 g.
- Protein: 10 g.
- Fiber: 3.2 g.
- Sugar: 10.7 g.

INGREDIENTS:

- **3 cups chickpeas (canned or cooked)**
- **1 large banana (ripe)**
- **½ cup chunky peanut butter (page 43)**
- **¼ cup peanuts (chopped)**
- **¼ cup maple syrup**
- **½ cup vegan protein powder (chocolate or banana flavor)**
- **1 tbsp. baking powder**
- **1 tbsp. ground flaxseed**
- **1 tbsp. vanilla extract**
- **½ tsp. cinnamon**
- **¼ tsp. nutmeg**
- **1 tbsp. cocoa nibs**
- **1 pinch of salt**

Total number of ingredients: 13

METHOD:

1. When using dry chickpeas, prepare 1 cup of dry chickpeas according to the method on page 31.
2. Preheat the oven to 375°F / 190°C.
3. Line a baking pan with parchment paper and set it aside.
4. Continue to add the cooked chickpeas and all the other ingredients—except the cocoa nibs—to a food processor. Pulse on low until the mixture is completely smooth, around 2-3 minutes.
5. Transfer the mixture to a large bowl and stir in the cocoa nibs.
6. Use a tablespoon to spoon the batter onto the baking pan, and then press down slightly on the top of the batter for even baking.
7. Place the pan with the spread batter in the oven and bake until golden, around 8-10 minutes.
8. Cool down, break into 8 pieces, and enjoy, share, or store!

Note: To get round cookies, you can also use your hands to roll the cookies into circular shapes before baking.

STORAGE INFORMATION:

Storage	Temperature	Expiration date	Preparation
Airtight container M/L	Fridge at 38 – 40°F or 3°C	4-5 days after preparation	Bring to room temperature
Airtight container M/L	Freezer at -1°F or -20°C	60 days after preparation	Thaw at room temperature

Tip: Chunky style peanut butter may cause the cookies to crumble. Add a tablespoon of extra peanut or palm oil to guarantee the best texture.

16. Chewy Almond Butter Balls

Serves: 2 | Prep Time: ~15 min |

Nutrition Information
(per serving)
- Calories: 329 kcal
- Carbs: 24.6 g.
- Fat: 16.5 g.
- Protein: 20.6 g.
- Fiber: 1 g.
- Sugar: 15.2 g.

INGREDIENTS:

- **2 tbsp. maple syrup**
- **½ cup vegan protein powder (vanilla or chocolate flavor)**
- **¼ cup almond butter**
- **1 tbsp. pure vanilla extract**
- **1 cup puffy rice cereal**
- **1 tbsp. carob chips**

Total number of ingredients: 6

METHOD:

1. Take a large bowl and thoroughly mix the maple syrup, protein powder, almond butter, and vanilla.
2. Microwave the bowl until the ingredients are heated through and the syrup and butter are melted, for about 40 seconds.
3. Add the puffy rice cereal and carob chips. Stir everything together evenly one more time.
4. Line a sheet pan with parchment paper, and using a spoon, scoop out the mixture and shape it into small-to-medium sized balls with your hands.
5. Press these balls firmly together to prevent crumbling and place them onto the pan with parchment paper.
6. Put the pan in the freezer for about 1 hour or leave in the fridge for 4 hours.
7. Enjoy the balls cold or thawed at room temperature. Alternatively, store them in a container or Ziploc bag to enjoy later.

STORAGE INFORMATION:

Storage	Temperature	Expiration date	Preparation
Airtight container M/L or Ziploc bag	Fridge at 38 – 40°F or 3°C	3-4 days after preparation	Enjoy chilled or at room temperature
Airtight container M/L or Ziploc bag	Freezer at -1°F or -20°C	60 days after preparation	Thaw in the fridge or at room temperature

Note: Substitute a gluten-free version of the puffy rice cereal in this easy snack.

Tip: Almond or peanut butter will hold these treats together better than creamier butters like cashew.

17. Hazelnut & Chocolate Bars

Nutrition Information
(per serving)
- Calories: 296 kcal
- Carbs: 21.3 g.
- Fat: 14.2 g.
- Protein: 20.6 g.
- Fiber: 3 g.
- Sugar: 12.7 g.

INGREDIENTS:

- **1 cup vegan chocolate protein powder**
- **¼ cup hazelnuts (chopped)**
- **¼ cup unsweetened cocoa powder**
- **⅓ cup almond milk**
- **¼ cup cashew butter**
- **3 tbsp. brown rice syrup**

Total number of ingredients: 6

METHOD:

1. In a large bowl, add the protein powder, cocoa, and hazelnuts; mix with a whisk to combine evenly.
2. Continue by adding the almond milk, cashew butter, and brown rice syrup; use the whisk or a small spatula to combine all ingredients thoroughly. Eventually the mixture should feel doughy and slightly sticky to the touch.
3. Lay out a sheet of parchment paper on a baking tray and place the dough in the middle. Press it out with your hands or a rolling pin until it's a ½-inch-thick square.
4. Put the baking tray in the fridge for 4 hours, or the freezer for 1½ hours.
5. Slice the chunk into 8 equal bars, and then serve and enjoy. Or, store for another day!

STORAGE INFORMATION:

Storage	Temperature	Expiration date	Preparation
Airtight container M/L or Ziploc bag	Fridge at 38 – 40°F or 3°C	4-5 days after preparation	
Airtight container M/L or Ziploc bag	Freezer at -1°F or -20°C	60 days after preparation	Thaw at room temperature

Note: Garnish with crushed hazelnuts or almonds for more crunch!

Tip: If the dough is too wet or sticky, add more cocoa or protein powder until you can handle it easily.

18. Nutty Blueberry Snack Squares

Serves: 6 | Prep Time: ~60 min |

Nutrition Information
(per serving)
- Calories: 246 kcal
- Carbs: 21.7 g.
- Fat: 13.1 g.
- Protein: 10.3 g.
- Fiber: 3 g.
- Sugar: 14.2 g.

INGREDIENTS:
- **1 cup raw almonds**
- **½ cup cashews**
- **½ cup puffy rice cereal**
- **½ cup vegan protein powder**
- **¼ cup dried blueberries**
- **¼ cup maple syrup**
- **1 pinch of salt**

Total number of ingredients: 7

METHOD:

1. Preheat the oven to 350°F / 175°C.
2. Line a square baking dish with parchment paper.
3. In a large bowl, add the almonds, cashews, rice cereal, blueberries, protein powder, and salt; stir well until all ingredients are evenly mixed.
4. Add the maple syrup and incorporate it thoroughly.
5. Spread the sticky mixture onto the parchment paper and pack it down tightly by using a spatula or your hands; be sure to press it into the corners as well.
6. Bake the mixture for 40-45 minutes, until stiff and the chunk begins to crisp.
7. Remove the baking dish from the oven, and after the dish has cooled, place it in the fridge for 30 minutes.
8. Cut the block into 12 even bars, and then serve, share, or store for another day!

STORAGE INFORMATION:

Storage	Temperature	Expiration date	Preparation
Airtight container M/L	Fridge at 38 – 40°F or 3°C	6-7 days after preparation	
Airtight container M/L	Freezer at -1°F or -20°C	60 days after preparation	Thaw at room temperature

Note: Dried cranberries, apricots, and/or cherries also make great additions to these bars.

Tip: Allow the bars to bake thoroughly. Otherwise they will fall apart once cooled.

19. Savory Sweet Lentil Bites

Serves: 8 | Prep Time: ~30 min |

Nutrition Information
(per serving)
- Calories: 264 kcal
- Carbs: 30.6 g.
- Fat: 12.4 g.
- Protein: 7.4 g.
- Fiber: 4.4 g.
- Sugar: 13.4 g.

INGREDIENTS:

- **2¼ cup green lentils (canned or cooked)**
- **½ tbsp. coconut oil**
- **½ tsp. cinnamon**
- **½ tsp. allspice**
- **1 pinch of salt**
- **1½ cup quick cooking oats**
- **¼ cup sunflower or pumpkin seeds**
- **¼ cup shredded coconut**
- **½ cup natural almond butter**
- **½ cup maple syrup**
- **¼ cup almonds (chopped or crushed)**

Total number of ingredients: 11

METHOD:

1. When using dry lentils, prepare the lentils according to the method on page 31.
2. Preheat the oven to 375°F / 190°C and line a baking pan with parchment paper.
3. Put the cooked lentils into a large bowl with the coconut oil, cinnamon, allspice, and salt; stir until everything is mixed well.
4. Place the lentil mixture on the baking pan and spread them out into a thin layer.
5. Bake them in the oven for 20 minutes, stirring once halfway through.
6. Remove the lentils from the oven and allow them to cool.
7. Mix the oats, seeds, shredded coconut, almond butter, maple syrup, and crushed almonds; stir well. Add the baked lentils and mix again until everything is well combined.
8. Roll the mixture into evenly-sized balls using a tablespoon or an ice cream scoop.
9. Refrigerate the balls on a plate in the fridge for 1 hour, or until the lentil balls have hardened. Serve, share, or store in a container for later.

STORAGE INFORMATION:

Storage	Temperature	Expiration date	Preparation
Airtight container M/L	Fridge at 38 – 40°F or 3°C	4-5 days after preparation	Consume chilled or bring to room temperature
Airtight container M/L	Freezer at -1°F or -20°C	60 days after preparation	Thaw in the fridge or at room temperature

Note: Add whatever seeds you have to pack these energy balls with even more nutrients.

Tip: Use brown or green lentils for this recipe. These types have the best texture for making balls.

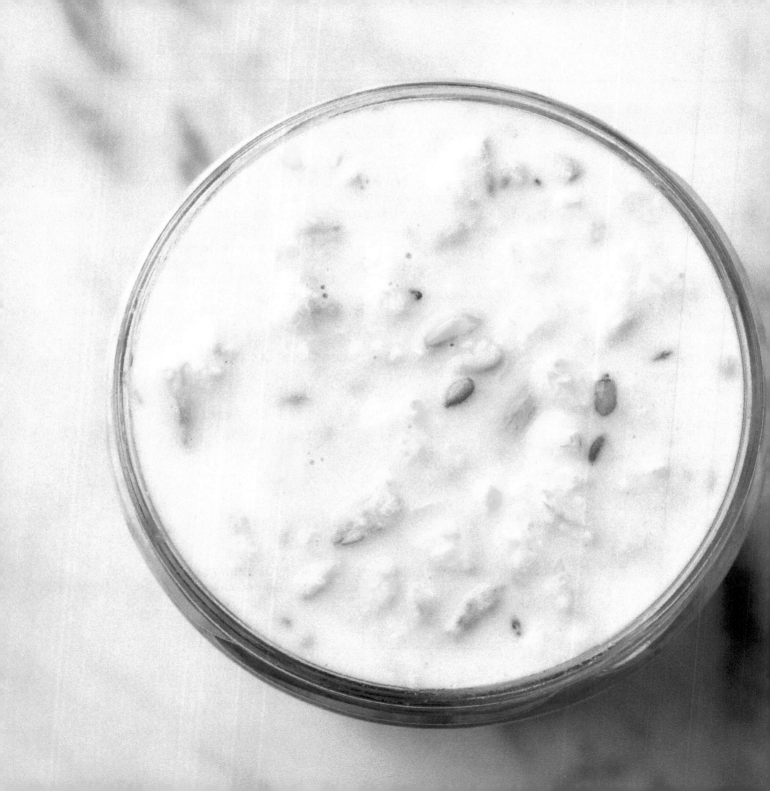

20. Overnight Cookie Dough Oats

Serves: 2 | Prep Time: ~10 min |

Nutrition Information
(per serving)
- Calories: 316 kcal
- Carbs: 22.7 g.
- Fat: 11.3 g.
- Protein: 30.7 g.
- Fiber: 4.2 g.
- Sugar: 1.3 g.

INGREDIENTS:

- ½ cup quick or rolled oats
- 1 tbsp. flaxseeds
- 2 scoops vegan protein powder (vanilla flavor)
- 1 cup almond milk (sweetened)
- 1 tbsp. peanut butter (page 43)
- Optional: 1 tbsp. maple syrup
- Optional: 1 tbsp. carob chips

Total number of ingredients: 7

METHOD:

1. Take a lidded bowl or jar and add the oats, flaxseed, protein powder, and almond milk.
2. Stir until everything is thoroughly combined and the mixture looks runny; if not, add a little more almond milk.
3. Blend in the peanut butter with a spoon until everything is mixed well.
4. Place or close the lid on the bowl or jar and transfer it to the refrigerator.
5. Allow the jar to sit overnight—or for at least five hours—so the flavors can set.
6. Serve the dough oats, and if desired, topped with the optional carob chips and a small cap of maple syrup.
7. Enjoy immediately, or store without the optional ingredients in an airtight container.

STORAGE INFORMATION:

Storage	Temperature	Expiration date	Preparation
Airtight container M/L	Fridge at 38 – 40°F or 3°C	3-4 days after preparation	Consume chilled
Airtight container M/L	Freezer at -1°F or -20°C	60 days after preparation	Thaw at room temperature

Note: Make sure the oats are certified gluten-free for a gluten-free snack!

Tip: You can substitute the peanut butter with almond or cashew butter. Replacing the butter will also result in a creamy thick mixture.

How to Use the Included Meal Plan

Preparing, or prepping, your meals is a real game changer. As in many of life's pursuits, habit and repetition will yield the best results. When it comes to prepping meals, it is best to develop a routine right from the start.

Every week, pick one or two days to dedicate 1-3 hours to cooking and prepping meals. It is recommended that you choose two days rather than one if storage space is limited, or you prefer to split cooking sessions up like this. Make sure to have all ingredients ready before you start cooking and prepare labels for each dish you're about to prep. Having staples such as rice, beans, and legumes prepared before a prepping session will make these cooking sessions even easier. These staples can easily be cooked and then frozen in large quantities. During a prepping session you can simply add the remaining ingredients in a recipe and save time. More about this in the chapter *'Prepping and Storing Food'* on page 156.

Keep a Schedule

Having a schedule in your agenda, notebook, or smartphone will help you remember what to eat on predetermined dates for each fueling meal and energizing snack. This schedule can simply be a copy of the meal plan you're going to use based on the 30-day meal plan in this book.

Label all the prepped dishes directly after cooking according to this schedule. Write both the recipe name and the date you will consume it on this label and add a matching note in your schedule. This will help you stick to your meal plan religiously and reduce stress.

The full 30-day meal plan would require you to prepare up to 25 recipes per week, but this is not necessary. **The best way to follow the plan is to pick two or three consecutive days of meals from the plan and repeat these a few times to create a weekly meal plan with fewer recipes that you can prepare in bulk.**

As long as you stick to the macro balances for each separate day of the meal plan, you are free to compose your own combination of days. You can select the recipes you enjoy the most, and at the same time, you'll only have to prepare four to eight dishes every week.

Macronutrients and Daily Calories

Each day of the 30-day meal plan guarantees the correct balance of macronutrients for your daily caloric intake. Taking your nutritional needs into consideration, you can easily determine the number of dish servings you'll need to prepare. As explained in the previous section, choose one, two, or more days from the meal plan and alternate these days throughout the week. Following a meal plan doesn't have to be boring; you can pick new days and adjust your preferences each new week for variety.

Each day in the included meal plan consists of five meals: breakfast, a snack, lunch, another snack, and dinner. The meal plan provides the number of servings needed for 1600, 1800, 2000, 2500, or 3000 calories per day. Remember that, depending on your bodyweight and goals, it's important to aim for a caloric deficit for weight loss, or a surplus of calories for muscle growth.

One gram of protein for each lean pound (1.5g/kg) of body weight per day is recommended for gaining muscle. In case your meals on a given day of the meal plan fail to deliver sufficient protein, you can supplement with one or more (plant-based) protein snacks or shakes. Note that these shakes have nutritional value and should be added to your daily caloric intake. As previously explained, tracking numbers is the key to progress, though small, unforeseen changes won't affect your progress right away, as long as it doesn't happen very often.

If you want to make any changes to the meal plan, **which is not recommended**, it's important to stick to the right daily balance of macronutrients. Every day, the combination of meals will deliver roughly 30-35% protein, 35-40% carbs, and 20-25% fats. If you want to replace a meal for a particular day because you don't like the recipe, you'll need to recalculate the total macronutrient proportions and calorie count. Make sure to swap the undesired meals with dishes that guarantee roughly the same nutritional value.

Tip: Use an app, Excel sheet, or a (digital) notepad to track your macronutrients. This will save you headaches and guarantee the right number of macros throughout the week. Some great apps include MyMacros+ (Android, iOS) and MyFitnessPal.

Ultimately, the goal is to find a meal prepping and eating routine that works for you. Always plan ahead of time to prevent having an empty fridge or freezer. Make meal prepping a habitual part of your life. Combine this with tracking your macronutrients and calories to guarantee the best results possible.

Grocery Lists and Shopping

*Note: Shopping lists for the included 30-day meal plan can be found on **https://tinyurl.com/grocerylists**.*

To optimize your trips to the grocery store, you'll benefit from creating custom shopping lists. Doing so requires you to list all ingredients required for the total amount of different recipes you plan to prep next, subtracting anything you already have in the pantry. Remember that you are free to prep either once or twice a week.

You can buy all the ingredients for the entire week in a single grocery shopping session or visit the store more than once. Taking fresh ingredients with a limited shelf life into consideration will be helpful. Veggies, fruits, and other ingredients that expire quickly might have to be bought more than once a week.

Tip: A seasoned meal prepper keeps the pantry stocked with nonperishables and keeps track of inventory, including products that are running low or nearing expiration date.

Make sure that on each trip to the grocery store, you bring a list and stick to it. Preparing a complete list will guarantee that you'll end up with all the ingredients required for your next cooking session. Buying only what's necessary will help you save money, prevent waste, and save you from breaking your head.

Save your lists to a cloud storage service like Google Drive so you can access them anytime, anywhere with a computer, tablet, or smartphone. This way, you'll always be able to access the shopping lists during your shopping trip. Alternatively, you can sign up for a grocery delivery service like Amazon Prime, Fresh, or Instacart. Apps for these services allow you to save shopping lists in the app. Using the services allow you to have all your groceries delivered without leaving the house.

*Note: Shopping lists for each week of the complete 30-day meal plan can be found at: **https://tinyurl.com/grocerylists***

Prepping and Storing Food

PREPPING INGREDIENTS

Preparing large amounts of staple foods and separate ingredients prior to prepping sessions will make you an even more efficient prepper. However, fresh vegetables and fruits are subject of a limited shelf life. In order to store these ingredients for longer periods of time, pre-treatment such as blanching will make it easier to freeze, dry, or can certain ingredients that otherwise expire fast.

Vegetables

Make sure to blanch vegetables with a high water content before freezing. Doing so will preserve their color, texture, and flavor. If these are not blanched prior to freezing, they will become limp, mushy or rubbery when thawed. Examples of water-rich vegetables include cucumber, lettuce, bean sprouts, cauliflower florets, zucchini, carrots, and tomatoes.

Blanching

Blanching helps to reduce quality loss of vegetables over time and is a very useful technique to preserve color, flavor, and nutritional value. It is done by rapidly heating and cooling vegetables to get rid of trapped air, inactivating enzymes, and to remove some of the water content.

Scald the vegetables in a blanching pot basket or sieve and submerge the vegetables in boiling water for a brief period, usually one or two minutes. After, the basket or sieve with its contents should be removed from the hot water and immediately transferred into a tub of cold water. Continue to drain the water and rinse the blanched vegetables with some fresh water before drying them off with paper towels and preparing them for storage in the freezer.

Fruits

Frozen fruits are great for cold and tasty smoothies. Prepping fruits upfront makes it super easy to grab a bag, transfer its contents into a blender and blend it with any additional ingredients into a quick smoothie.

Fruits that freeze well include apples, avocados, pears,

kiwis, oranges, grapefruit, lemons, limes, peaches, plums, nectarines, bananas, raspberries, blackberries, watermelon, honeydew melons, cantaloupe, apricots, grapes, mangoes, cherries, strawberries, blueberries, raisins, currants, cranberries, and figs. Note that most of these fruits can also be bought pre-cut, peeled and frozen.

OTHER INGREDIENTS TO FREEZE

Fresh herbs and spices such as lemon balm, mint, basil, chives, oregano, thyme, and cumin are freezer-friendly. However, most of them are also sold in dried from, which makes it a lot easier to store them. To freeze fresh herbs, remove the leaves from the stems and allow the herbs to dry out before freezing them. This is best done in a Ziploc bag. Alternatively, herbs can be mixed with water or oil before being transferred into the freezer. Freezing your own herbs will result in semi-fresh herbs that have a different taste profile compared to their store-bought, dried ingredients.

Freezer tips

The freezer is one of the most useful devices for the meal prepper. There are some things to keep in mind when using it.

- Regularly clean out the freezer.
- Always allow freshly cooked meals to cool down to room temperature and/or use the refrigerator to cool the meals completely before freezing in order to preserve flavor and texture.
- A filled freezer is more economical as the air in it will be kept cold more easily. Don't overload the freezer, which will be preventing the air from circulating.
- Try to open the freezer door only for storing new or taking out dishes or ingredients. This will save energy and prevent the food that's already inside from defrosting.

Heating Stored Food

Some of the prepped dishes require reheating before eating. Here are these some of the best ways to do so:

1) **Stove**: place your food in a saucepan and heat it thoroughly while occasionally stirring.

2) **Oven**: place the food in a heat resistant container or spread it out on a baking dish. Make sure not to set the oven at a high temperature to prevent the food from being burned.

3) **Microwave:** a quick way to reheat food that will save you a lot of time. Make sure to use containers that are microwave safe.

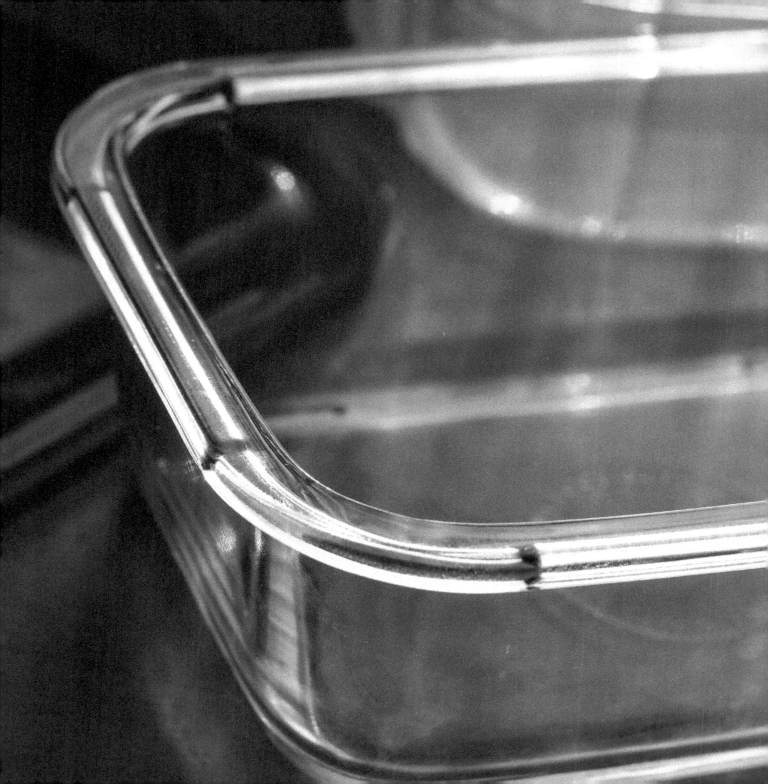

Containers for Storing Food

Common food-storing methods include:

1. Refrigerating and freezing – storing food at lower temperatures will maintain its freshness and nutritious value for longer.
2. Drying food – dehydrating foods (sun drying, air-drying, oven drying, and smoking) keeps food from going bad as bacteria cannot thrive without water.
3. Canning – sealing food in airtight containers also stops bacteria or fungi from multiplying, as they require oxygen.
4. Pickling – storing food in vinegar and salt mixtures is another common method for preserving fresh food.

When choosing a container for storing food, factors such as portion size, storage time, space available in the fridge/freezer, and dimensions should be taken into consideration. Knowing the amount of available storage space will guarantee that you are not wasting ingredients and time. It will also prevent buying things you cannot keep.

Multiple compartment containers with different, separate sections will help to preserve taste and texture of prepped meals. As the different elements of a dish are being kept separate, the aesthetics are also improved, which will result in a tastier-looking meal.

Make sure that the containers you buy are free from bisphenol (BPA). Transparent containers will help you to identify your meals more easily when they are stacked, and labels are hidden from sight. For longer storage periods, containers with a vacuum seal may also be useful.

Common food storage containers:

1. Polycarbonate containers: transparent, shatter-proof, and usually with airtight lids.
2. Polypropylene containers: temperature-resistant, stackable, and BPA-free.
3. Stainless steel containers: temperature-resistant but not suitable for the microwave.
4. Glass containers: high-quality, easy to keep clean, temperature-resistant, stackable, and suitable for the microwave.
5. Ingredient bins: for bulk foods like grains.

Food labeling is very important for organizational purposes. Labeling every container before it goes into the fridge or freezer will make meal prepping and following a meal plan easy.

Labeling ingredient bins and organizing your pantry properly will help you prevent ingredients from running out. Labeling can help you run an organized, efficient, and healthy kitchen.

Label tips:

Freezing: use blank food labels that are printed professionally and freezer-friendly. These labels won't come off your packaging and low temperatures do not affect the readability.

It is important to include:

- The date of cooking/prepping the dish
- Name of the meal
- The (estimated) expiration date
- The day of the meal plan for which the dish has been prepared
- Optional: calories and macros for each portion (see recipe or meal plan)

30-Day Meal Plan

Week 1: Meal Plan

Make sure to read the chapter 'Using the 14-day meal plan' before using this meal plan!

Shopping lists for each week of the complete 30-day meal plan can be found at: **https://tinyurl.com/grocerylists**

MEAL PLAN	MONDAY	
BREAKFAST	ALMOND EXPLOSION *(page 65)*	1 SERVING
A.M. SNACK	HAZELNUT & CHOCOLATE BARS *(page 149)*	1 SERVING
LUNCH	LENTIL. LEMON AND MUSHROOM SALAD *(page 67)*	2 SERVINGS
P.M. SNACK	SUNFLOWER PROTEIN BARS *(page 143)*	1 SERVING
DINNER	BLACK BEAN AND QUINOA BURGERS *(page 111)*	1 SERVING

CARBS	FAT	PROTEIN	CALORIES	SERVINGS	SERVINGS	SERVINGS	SERVINGS
29.5 g.	15 g.	25.4 g.	355 Kcal	1	1	2	2
21.3 g.	14.2 g.	20.6 g.	296 Kcal	1	1	1	2
56.2 g.	19.2 g.	31.6 g.	524 Kcal	2	2	2	2
21.9 g.	6.8 g.	9.6 g.	188 Kcal	1	1	2	3
40.5 g.	10.6 g.	9.5 g.	200 Kcal	2	3	3	3
169.4 g.	**65.8 g.**	**96.7 g.**	**1563 Kcal**	**1763 Kcal**	**1963 Kcal**	**2506 Kcal**	**2990 Kcal**

MEAL PLAN		TUESDAY			
BREAKFAST	POWERHOUSE PROTEIN SHAKE *(page 61)*				1 SERVING
A.M. SNACK	NO-BAKE ALMOND-RICE TREATS *(page 142)*				1 SERVING
LUNCH	SWEET POTATO AND BLACK BEAN PROTEIN SALAD *(page 68)*				1 SERVING
P.M. SNACK	OVERNIGHT COOKIE DOUGH OATS *(page 153)*				1 SERVING
DINNER	STUFFED INDIAN EGGPLANT *(page 107)*				3 SERVINGS

CARBS	FAT	PROTEIN	CALORIES	SERVINGS	SERVINGS	SERVINGS	SERVINGS
30 g.	3.5 g.	26.3 g.	257 Kcal	2	2	2	2
13.2 g.	11.2 g.	9.3 g.	191 Kcal	1	2	2	3
48.8 g.	14.5 g.	11.4 g.	370 Kcal	1	1	2	2
22.7 g.	11.3 g.	30.7 g.	316 Kcal	1	1	1	2
54.9 g.	18 g.	13.2 g.	435 Kcal	3	3	4	4
169.6 g.	**58.5 g.**	**90.9 g.**	**1569 Kcal**	**1826 Kcal**	**2017 Kcal**	**2532 Kcal**	**3039 Kcal**

MEAL PLAN		WEDNESDAY			
BREAKFAST	ALMOND PROTEIN SHAKE *(page 63)*				1 SERVING
A.M. SNACK	MATCHA ENERGY BALLS *(page 133)*				1 SERVING
LUNCH	SOUTHWEST STYLE SALAD *(page 73)*				1 SERVING
P.M. SNACK	LEMON LIME PIE BARS *(page 134)*				1 SERVING
DINNER	SWEET POTATO SUSHI *(page 116)*				1 SERVING

CARBS	FAT	PROTEIN	CALORIES	SERVINGS	SERVINGS	SERVINGS	SERVINGS
15.2 g.	17 g.	31.6 g.	340 Kcal	1	1	2	2
21.3 g.	21.2 g.	14.6 g.	335 Kcal	1	1	1	2
51 g.	16.8 g.	11.2 g.	397 Kcal	1½	2	2	2
34.9 g.	10.7 g.	8.9 g.	272 Kcal	1	1	1	1
39.2 g.	10.3 g.	10.3 g.	290 Kcal	1	1	1½	2
161.6 g.	**76 g.**	**76.6 g.**	**1634 Kcal**	**1832 Kcal**	**2030 Kcal**	**2515 Kcal**	**2995 Kcal**

MEAL PLAN		THURSDAY	
BREAKFAST	CRANBERRY PROTEIN SHAKE *(page 59)*		1 SERVING
A.M. SNACK	MOCHA CHOCOLATE BROWNIE BARS *(page 144)*		2 SERVINGS
LUNCH	CUBAN TEMPEH BUDDHA BOWL *(page 117)*		1 SERVING
P.M. SNACK	NUTTY BLUEBERRY SNACK SQUARES *(page 150)*		1 SERVING
DINNER	TOFU CACCIATORE *(page 97)*		1 SERVING

CARBS	FAT	PROTEIN	CALORIES	SERVINGS	SERVINGS	SERVINGS	SERVINGS
19.9 g.	16.8 g.	23.6 g.	325 Kcal	1	1	1	1
34.6 g.	7.6 g.	54.6 g.	416 Kcal	3	4	4	5
27.4 g.	18.3 g.	17.6 g.	343 Kcal	1	1	1	1
21.7 g.	13.1 g.	10.3 g.	246 Kcal	1	1	2	2
33.7 g.	9.5 g.	13.6 g.	274 Kcal	1	1	2	3
137.3 g.	**65.3 g.**	**119.7 g.**	**1604 Kcal**	**1812 Kcal**	**2020 Kcal**	**2540 Kcal**	**3022 Kcal**

MEAL PLAN		FRIDAY	
BREAKFAST	AVOCADO-CHIA PROTEIN SHAKE *(page 62)*		1 SERVING
A.M. SNACK	CRANBERRY VANILLA PROTEIN BARS *(page 145)*		1 SERVING
LUNCH	SHAVED BRUSSEL SPROUT SALAD *(page 74)*		1 SERVING
P.M. SNACK	SPICY CHICKPEA POPPERS *(page 129)*		1 SERVING
DINNER	HIGH PROTEIN BLACK BEAN DIP *(page 135)*		1 SERVING

CARBS	FAT	PROTEIN	CALORIES	SERVINGS	SERVINGS	SERVINGS	SERVINGS
16.6 g.	21.4 g.	30.1 g.	379 Kcal	1	1	1	1
22.9 g.	9.6 g.	16.1 g.	243 Kcal	1	2	3	3½
45.3 g.	18.7 g.	11.5 g.	396 Kcal	1	1	1	2
21.5 g.	7.8 g.	9.1 g.	192 Kcal	2	2	3	3
63 g.	6.6 g.	21.3 g.	398 Kcal	1	1	1	1
169.3 g.	**64.1 g.**	**88.1 g.**	**1608 Kcal**	**1800 Kcal**	**2043 Kcal**	**2478 Kcal**	**2995 Kcal**

Make sure to read the chapter 'Using the 14-day meal plan' before using this meal plan!

Shopping lists for each week of the complete 30-day meal plan can be found at: **https://tinyurl.com/grocerylists**

MEAL PLAN	MONDAY	
BREAKFAST	BANANA PROTEIN PUNCH *(page 66)*	1 SERVING
A.M. SNACK	CHOCOLATE. QUINOA AND ZUCCHINI MUFFINS *(page 127)*	1 SERVING
LUNCH	COLORFUL PROTEIN POWER SALAD *(page 75)*	1 SERVING
P.M. SNACK	GLUTEN-FREE ENERGY CRACKERS *(page 125)*	1 SERVING
DINNER	MANGO-TEMPEH WRAPS *(page 83)*	1 SERVING

CARBS	FAT	PROTEIN	CALORIES	SERVINGS	SERVINGS	SERVINGS	SERVINGS
23.3 g.	10 g.	20.2 g.	264 Kcal	1	1	1	1
30.4 g.	19.4 g.	14.2 g.	354 Kcal	1	1	1	1
64.8 g.	15.5 g.	22.3 g.	487 Kcal	1	1	2	2
10.3 g.	15.6 g.	6.9 g.	209 Kcal	2	2	2	3
31.3 g.	7.8 g.	15.7 g.	259 Kcal	1	2	2	3
160.1 g.	**68.3 g.**	**79.3 g.**	**1573 Kcal**	**1782 Kcal**	**2041 Kcal**	**2528 Kcal**	**2996 Kcal**

MEAL PLAN		TUESDAY					
BREAKFAST	ALMOND PROTEIN SHAKE *(page 63)*				1 SERVING		
A.M. SNACK	SUNFLOWER PROTEIN BARS *(page 143)*				1 SERVING		
LUNCH	CREAMY SQUASH PIZZA *(page 84)*				1 SERVING		
P.M. SNACK	CHEVY ALMOND BUTTER BALLS *(page 148)*				1 SERVING		
DINNER	EDAMAME AND GINGER CITRUS SALAD *(page 76)*				1 SERVING		

CARBS	FAT	PROTEIN	CALORIES	SERVINGS	SERVINGS	SERVINGS	SERVINGS
15.2 g.	17 g.	31.6 g.	340 Kcal	1	1	2	2
21.9 g.	6.8 g.	9.6 g.	188 Kcal	2	3	4	5
62.5 g.	8.6 g.	18.4 g.	401 Kcal	1	1	1	1
24.6 g.	16.5 g.	20.6 g.	329 Kcal	1	1	1	2
38.9 g.	11.4 g.	14.4 g.	316 Kcal	1	1	1	1
163.1 g.	**60.3 g.**	**94.6 g.**	**1574 Kcal**	**1762 Kcal**	**1950 Kcal**	**2478 Kcal**	**2995 Kcal**

MEAL PLAN		WEDNESDAY					
BREAKFAST	CRANBERRY PROTEIN SHAKE *(page 59)*				1 SERVING		
A.M. SNACK	OVERNIGHT COOKIE DOUGH OATS *(page 153)*				1 SERVING		
LUNCH	SUPER SUMMER SALAD *(page 69)*				1 SERVING		
P.M. SNACK	NUTTY BLUEBERRY SNACK SQUARES *(page 150)*				1 SERVING		
DINNER	SWEET POTATO CHILI *(page 113)*				2 SERVINGS		

CARBS	FAT	PROTEIN	CALORIES	SERVINGS	SERVINGS	SERVINGS	SERVINGS
19.9 g.	16.8 g.	23.6 g.	325 Kcal	1	1	2	2
22.7 g.	11.3 g.	30.7 g.	316 Kcal	1	1	1	2
33.3 g.	20.8 g.	12.3 g.	371 Kcal	1	1	1	1
21.7 g.	13.1 g.	10.3 g.	246 Kcal	1	2	2	2
31.4 g.	17 g.	17.2 g.	346 Kcal	3	3	4	5
129 g.	**79 g.**	**94.1 g.**	**1604 Kcal**	**1777 Kcal**	**2023 Kcal**	**2521 Kcal**	**3010 Kcal**

MEAL PLAN			THURSDAY				
BREAKFAST	AVOCADO-CHIA PROTEIN SHAKE *(page 62)*				1 SERVING		
A.M. SNACK	PEANUT BUTTER AND BANANA COOKIES *(page 147)*				1 SERVING		
LUNCH	MUSHROOM PHO *(page 79)*				1 SERVING		
P.M. SNACK	ALMOND AND DATE PROTEIN BARS *(page 125)*				1 SERVING		
DINNER	RUBY RED ROOTBEET BURGER *(page 81)*				2 SERVINGS		

CARBS	FAT	PROTEIN	CALORIES	SERVINGS	SERVINGS	SERVINGS	SERVINGS
16.6 g.	21.4 g.	30.1 g.	379 Kcal	1	1	1	1
20.2 g.	11 g.	10 g.	220 Kcal	1	1	2	2
57.3 g.	9.1 g.	17.8 g.	383 Kcal	1	1	1	2
15.6 g.	17.4 g.	10.5 g.	261 Kcal	2	2	3	3
46.4 g.	9.8 g.	11.2 g.	318 Kcal	2	3	3	4
156.1 g.	**68.7 g.**	**79.6 g.**	**1561 Kcal**	**1822 Kcal**	**1981 Kcal**	**2462 Kcal**	**3004 Kcal**

MEAL PLAN			FRIDAY				
BREAKFAST	ALMOND AND DATE PROTEIN BARS *(page 125)*				1 SERVING		
A.M. SNACK	TROPICAL PROTEIN SMOOTHIE *(page 58)*				1 SERVING		
LUNCH	LASAGNA FUNGO *(page 85)*				1 SERVING		
P.M. SNACK	SAVORY SWEET LENTIL BITES *(page 151)*				1 SERVING		
DINNER	STACKED N' SPICY PORTOBELLO BURGERS *(page 125)*				1 SERVING		

CARBS	FAT	PROTEIN	CALORIES	SERVINGS	SERVINGS	SERVINGS	SERVINGS
15.6 g.	17.4 g.	10.5 g.	261 Kcal	1	1	2	2
44.4 g.	6.7 g.	27.9 g.	350 Kcal	1	1	1	1
38 g.	9.2 g.	14.2 g.	292 Kcal	1	1	1	1
30.6 g.	12.4 g.	7.4 g.	264 Kcal	1	1	2	2
48.9 g.	16 g.	20.5 g.	421 Kcal	1½	2	2	3
177.5 g.	**61.7 g.**	**80.5 g.**	**1588 Kcal**	**1798 Kcal**	**2009 Kcal**	**2534 Kcal**	**2955 Kcal**

Make sure to read the chapter 'Using the 14-day meal plan' before using this meal plan!

*Shopping lists for each week of the complete 30-day meal plan can be found at: **https://tinyurl.com/grocerylists***

MEAL PLAN	MONDAY	
BREAKFAST	CINNAMON APPLE PROTEIN SMOOTHIE *(page 57)*	1 SERVING
A.M. SNACK	LEMON LIME PIE BARS *(page 134)*	1 SERVING
LUNCH	PORTOBELLO BURRITOS *(page 99)*	2 SERVINGS
P.M. SNACK	LENTIL RADISH SALAD *(page 71)*	1 SERVING
DINNER	MUSHROOM MADNESS STROGANOFF *(page 101)*	1 SERVING

CARBS	FAT	PROTEIN	CALORIES	SERVINGS	SERVINGS	SERVINGS	SERVINGS
21.7 g.	10.3 g.	48.5 g.	373 Kcal	1	1	1	1
34.9 g.	10.7 g.	8.9 g.	272 Kcal	1	1	1	2
68 g.	18.4 g.	10.2 g.	478 Kcal	2	2	4	4
25.3 g.	10.7 g.	12.4 g.	247 Kcal	2	2	2	2
27.8 g.	6.5 g.	7.6 g.	200 Kcal	1	2	2	3
177.7 g.	**56.6 g.**	**87.6 g.**	**1570 Kcal**	**1817 Kcal**	**2017 Kcal**	**2495 Kcal**	**2967 Kcal**

MEAL PLAN				TUESDAY			
BREAKFAST	CANDIED PROTEIN TRAIL MIX *(page 141)*						1 SERVING
A.M. SNACK	HIGH PROTEIN CAKE BATTER SMOOTHIE *(page 137)*						1 SERVING
LUNCH	CREAMY SQUASH PIZZA *(page 84)*						1 SERVING
P.M. SNACK	CHOCOLATE .QUINOA AND ZUCCHINI MUFFINS *(page 127)*						1 SERVING
DINNER	SWEET AND SOUR TOFU *(page 89)*						1 SERVING

CARBS	FAT	PROTEIN	CALORIES	SERVINGS	SERVINGS	SERVINGS	SERVINGS
19.5 g.	28 g.	14 g.	387 Kcal	1	1	1	1
27.2 g.	7.6 g.	16 g.	241 Kcal	1	1	2	3
62.5 g.	8.6 g.	18.4 g.	401 Kcal	1½	2	2	2
304 g.	19.4 g.	14.2 g.	354 Kcal	1	1	1	1
24.3 g.	11.5 g.	8.8 g.	236 Kcal	1	1	2	3
437.5 g.	**75.1 g.**	**71.4 g.**	**1619 Kcal**	**1819 Kcal**	**2020 Kcal**	**2497 Kcal**	**2974 Kcal**

MEAL PLAN				WEDNESDAY			
BREAKFAST	CHEWY ALMOND BUTTER BALLS *(page 148)*						1 SERVING
A.M. SNACK	GLUTEN FREE ENERGY CRACKERS *(page 125)*						1 SERVING
LUNCH	MOROCCAN EGGPLANT STEW *(page 103)*						1 SERVING
P.M. SNACK	MOCHA CHOCOLATE BROWNIE BARS *(page 144)*						1 SERVING
DINNER	TACO TEMPEH SALAD *(page 77)*						1 SERVING

CARBS	FAT	PROTEIN	CALORIES	SERVINGS	SERVINGS	SERVINGS	SERVINGS
24.6 g.	16.5 g.	20.6 g.	329 Kcal	1	1	1	2
10.3 g.	15.6 g.	6.9 g.	209 Kcal	1	2	2	3
80.5 g.	2.7 g.	17.7 g.	417 Kcal	1	1	1	1
17.3 g.	3.8 g.	27.3 g.	213 Kcal	2	2	2	2
36.3 g.	23 g.	22.4 g.	441 Kcal	1	1	2	2
169 g.	**61.6 g.**	**94.9 g.**	**1609 Kcal**	**1822 Kcal**	**2031 Kcal**	**2472 Kcal**	**3010 Kcal**

MEAL PLAN			THURSDAY				
BREAKFAST		BANANA PROTEIN PUNCH *(page 66)*					1 SERVING
A.M. SNACK		SUNFLOWER PROTEIN BARS *(page 143)*					1 SERVING
LUNCH		REFINED RATATOUILLE *(page 105)*					1 SERVING
P.M. SNACK		SPICY CHICKPEA POPPERS *(page 129)*					1 SERVING
DINNER		BARBECUED GREENS AND GRITS *(page 108)*					1 SERVING

CARBS	FAT	PROTEIN	CALORIES	SERVINGS	SERVINGS	SERVINGS	SERVINGS
23.3 g.	10 g.	20.2 g.	264 Kcal	1	1	1	2
21.9 g.	6.8 g.	9.6 g.	188 Kcal	1	2	2	3
61.2 g.	24.3 g.	23.7 g.	558 Kcal	1	1	2	2
21.5 g.	7.8 g.	9.1 g.	192 Kcal	2	2	2	2
39.3 g.	17.6 g.	19.7 g.	394 Kcal	1	1	1	1
167.2 g.	**66.5 g.**	**82.3 g.**	**1596 Kcal**	**1788 Kcal**	**1976 Kcal**	**2534 Kcal**	**2986 Kcal**

MEAL PLAN			FRIDAY				
BREAKFAST		AVOCADO CHIA PROTEIN SHAKE *(page 62)*					1 SERVING
A.M. SNACK		CRANBERRY VANILLA PROTEIN BARS *(page 145)*					1 SERVING
LUNCH		ROASTED ALMOND PROTEIN SALAD *(page 70)*					2 SERVINGS
P.M. SNACK		LEMON LIME PIE BARS *(page 134)*					1 SERVING
DINNER		SWEET POTATO QUESADILLAS *(page 93)*					1 SERVING

CARBS	FAT	PROTEIN	CALORIES	SERVINGS	SERVINGS	SERVINGS	SERVINGS
16.6 g.	21.4 g.	30.1 g.	379 Kcal	1	1	1	1
22.9 g.	9.6 g.	16.1 g.	243 Kcal	1	1	1	2
50 g.	14.8 g.	20 g.	412 Kcal	3	4	5	6
34.9 g.	10.7 g.	8.9 g.	272 Kcal	1	1	2	2
54.8 g.	7.5 g.	10.6 g.	329 Kcal	1	1	1	1
179.2 g.	**64 g.**	**85.7 g.**	**1635 Kcal**	**1841 Kcal**	**2047 Kcal**	**2525 Kcal**	**2974 Kcal**

Make sure to read the chapter 'Using the 14-day meal plan' before using this meal plan!

Shopping lists for each week of the complete 30-day meal plan can be found at: ***https://tinyurl.com/grocerylists***

MEAL PLAN	MONDAY	
BREAKFAST	CINNAMON APPLE PROTEIN SMOOTHIE *(page 57)*	1 SERVING
A.M. SNACK	NUTTY BLUEBERRY SNACK SQUARES *(page 150)*	1 SERVING
LUNCH	STUFFED INDIAN EGGPLANT *(page 107)*	3 SERVINGS
P.M. SNACK	SAVORY SWEET LENTIL BITES *(page 151)*	1 SERVING
DINNER	TERIYAKI TOFU WRAPS *(page 94)*	1 SERVING

CARBS	FAT	PROTEIN	CALORIES	SERVINGS	SERVINGS	SERVINGS	SERVINGS
21.7 g.	10.3 g.	48.5 g.	373 Kcal	1	1	1	1
21.7 g.	13.1 g.	10.3 g.	246 Kcal	2	2	3	3
54.9 g.	18 g.	13.2 g.	435 Kcal	3	4	4	4
30.6 g.	12.4 g.	7.4 g.	264 Kcal	1	1	2	3
20.5 g.	15.4 g.	12.1 g.	259 Kcal	1	1	1	2
149.4 g.	**69.2 g.**	**91.5 g.**	**1577 Kcal**	**1823 Kcal**	**1968 Kcal**	**2478 Kcal**	**3001 Kcal**

MEAL PLAN		TUESDAY	
BREAKFAST	MOCHA CHOCOLATE BROWNIE BARS *(page 144)*		1 SERVING
A.M. SNACK	OVERNIGHT COOKIE DOUGH OATS *(page 153)*		1 SERVING
LUNCH	SATAY TEMPEH WITH CAULIFLOWER RICE *(page 91)*		1 SERVING
P.M. SNACK	BANANA PROTEIN PUNCH *(page 66)*		1 SERVING
DINNER	TEX-MEX TOFU AND BEANS *(page 95)*		1 SERVING

CARBS	FAT	PROTEIN	CALORIES	SERVINGS	SERVINGS	SERVINGS	SERVINGS
17.3 g.	3.8 g.	27.3 g.	213 Kcal	1	1	1	2
22.7 g.	11.3 g.	30.7 g.	316 Kcal	1	1	1	1
31.7 g.	33 g.	27.6 g.	531 Kcal	1	1	2	2
23.3 g.	10 g.	20.2 g.	264 Kcal	1	1	1	2
27.8 g.	14 g.	12.7 g.	315 Kcal	1½	2	2	2
122.8 g.	**72.1 g.**	**118.5 g.**	**1639 Kcal**	**1796 Kcal**	**1953 Kcal**	**2484 Kcal**	**2961 Kcal**

MEAL PLAN		WEDNESDAY	
BREAKFAST	ALMOND EXPLOSION *(page 65)*		1 SERVING
A.M. SNACK	MATCHA ENERGY BALLS *(page 133)*		1 SERVING
LUNCH	STUFFED SWEET POTATOES *(page 90)*		1 SERVING
P.M. SNACK	SUNFLOWER PROTEIN BARS *(page 143)*		1 SERVING
DINNER	RED BEANS AND RICE *(page 125)*		1 SERVING

CARBS	FAT	PROTEIN	CALORIES	SERVINGS	SERVINGS	SERVINGS	SERVINGS
29.5 g.	15 g.	25.4 g.	355 Kcal	1	1	1	1
21.3 g.	21.2 g.	14.6 g.	335 Kcal	1	1	1	1
55.7 g.	17.1 g.	20.7 g.	498 Kcal	1	1	2	3
21.9 g.	6.8 g.	9.6 g.	188 Kcal	1	2	2	2
32.3 g.	8.3 g.	7.9 g.	235 Kcal	2	2	2	2
160.7 g.	**68.4 g.**	**78.2 g.**	**1611 Kcal**	**1846 Kcal**	**2034 Kcal**	**2532 Kcal**	**3030 Kcal**

MEAL PLAN				THURSDAY			
BREAKFAST	CRANBERRY PROTEIN SHAKE *(page 59)*						1 SERVING
A.M. SNACK	HAZELNUT AND CHOCOLATE PROTEIN BARS *(page 149)*						1 SERVING
LUNCH	COCONUT TOFU CURRY *(page 119)*						1 SERVING
P.M. SNACK	ALMOND AND DATE PROTEIN BARS *(page 125)*						1 SERVING
DINNER	TAHINI FALAFELS *(page 121)*						1 SERVING

CARBS	FAT	PROTEIN	CALORIES	SERVINGS	SERVINGS	SERVINGS	SERVINGS
19.9 g.	16.8 g.	23.6 g.	325 Kcal	1	1	1	1
21.3 g.	14.2 g.	20.6 g.	296 Kcal	1	1	1	2
38.7 g.	23 g.	21.8 g.	449 Kcal	1	1	2	2
15.6 g.	17.4 g.	10.5 g.	261 Kcal	1	2	2	2
28 g.	7.3 g.	10.5 g.	220 Kcal	2	2	2	3
123.5 g.	**78.7 g.**	**87 g.**	**1551 Kcal**	**1771 Kcal**	**2032 Kcal**	**2481 Kcal**	**2997 Kcal**

MEAL PLAN				FRIDAY			
BREAKFAST	ALMOND AND PROTEIN SHAKE *(page 63)*						1 SERVING
A.M. SNACK	GLUTEN-FREE ENERGY CRACKERS *(page 125)*						1 SERVING
LUNCH	HIGH PROTEIN BLACK BEAN DIP *(page 135)*						1 SERVING
P.M. SNACK	LEMON LIME PIE BARS *(page 134)*						1 SERVING
DINNER	BAKED ENCHILADA BOWLS *(page 124)*						1 SERVING

CARBS	FAT	PROTEIN	CALORIES	SERVINGS	SERVINGS	SERVINGS	SERVINGS
15.2 g.	17 g.	31.6 g.	340 Kcal	1	1	1	1
10.3 g.	15.6 g.	6.9 g.	209 Kcal	2	2	2	3
63 g.	6.6 g.	21.3 g.	398 Kcal	1	1	1	1
34.9 g.	10.7 g.	8.9 g.	272 Kcal	1	1½	2	3
34.6 g.	27.1 g.	15.6 g.	417 Kcal	1	1	2	2
158 g.	**77 g.**	**84.3 g.**	**1636 Kcal**	**1845 Kcal**	**1981 Kcal**	**2534 Kcal**	**3015 Kcal**

Week 5: Meal Plan

Make sure to read the chapter 'Using the 14-day meal plan' before using this meal plan!

*Shopping lists for each week of the complete 30-day meal plan can be found at: **https://tinyurl.com/grocerylists***

MEAL PLAN	MONDAY	
BREAKFAST	CANDIED PROTEIN TRAIL MIX *(page 141)*	1 SERVING
A.M. SNACK	NO-BAKE ALMOND RICE TREATS *(page 142)*	1 SERVING
LUNCH	GREEN THAI CURRY *(page 123)*	1 SERVING
P.M. SNACK	CRANBERRY VANILLA PROTEIN BARS *(page 145)*	1 SERVING
DINNER	MOROCCAN EGGPLANT STEW *(page 103)*	1 SERVING

CARBS	FAT	PROTEIN	CALORIES	SERVINGS	SERVINGS	SERVINGS	SERVINGS
19.5 g.	28 g.	14 g.	387 Kcal	1	1	1	1
13.2 g.	11.2 g.	9.3 g.	191 Kcal	1	2	3	4
35.6 g.	14.9 g.	12.5 g.	327 Kcal	1	1	2	3
22.9 g.	9.6 g.	16.1 g.	243 Kcal	2	2	2	2
80.5 g.	2.7 g.	17.7 g.	417 Kcal	1	1	1	1
171.7 g.	**66.4 g.**	**69.6 g.**	**1565 Kcal**	**1808 Kcal**	**1999 Kcal**	**2517 Kcal**	**3032 Kcal**

MEAL PLAN				TUESDAY			
BREAKFAST	OATMEAL PROTEIN MIX *(page 64)*						1 SERVING
A.M. SNACK	MOCHA CHOCOLATE BROWNIE BARS *(page 144)*						1 SERVING
LUNCH	STUFFED SWEET POTATOES *(page 90)*						1 SERVING
P.M. SNACK	PEANUT BUTTER AND BANANA COOKIES *(page 147)*						1 SERVING
DINNER	SOUTHWEST STUFFED AVOCADO BOWLS *(page 139)*						1 SERVING

CARBS	FAT	PROTEIN	CALORIES	SERVINGS	SERVINGS	SERVINGS	SERVINGS
24.7 g.	9 g.	29.3 g.	298 Kcal	1	1	1	2
17.3 g.	3.8 g.	27.3 g.	213 Kcal	1	2	2	2
55.7 g.	17.7 g.	20.7 g.	498 Kcal	1	1	2	2
20.2 g.	11 g.	10 g.	220 Kcal	2	2	2	3
32.6 g.	20 g.	10 g.	351 Kcal	1	1	1	1
150.5 g.	**61.5 g.**	**97.3 g.**	**1580 Kcal**	**1800 Kcal**	**2013 Kcal**	**2511 Kcal**	**3029 Kcal**

MEAL PLAN				WEDNESDAY			
BREAKFAST	BANANA PROTEIN PUNCH *(page 66)*						2 SERVINGS
A.M. SNACK	ALMOND AND DATE PROTEIN BARS *(page 125)*						1 SERVING
LUNCH	MUSHROOM MADNESS STROGANOFF *(page 101)*						1 SERVING
P.M. SNACK	EDAMAME AND GINGER CITRUS SALAD *(page 76)*						1 SERVING
DINNER	VEGAN FRIENDLY FAJITAS *(page 98)*						1 SERVING

CARBS	FAT	PROTEIN	CALORIES	SERVINGS	SERVINGS	SERVINGS	SERVINGS
46.6 g.	20 g.	40.4 g.	528 Kcal	2	2	2	2
15.6 g.	17.4 g.	10.5 g.	261 Kcal	2	2	2	2
27.8 g.	6.5 g.	7.6 g.	200 Kcal	1	2	3	4
38.9 g.	11.4 g.	14.4 g.	316 Kcal	1	1	2	2
27.7 g.	14 g.	6.8 g.	264 Kcal	1	1	1	1
156.6 g.	**69.3 g.**	**79.7 g.**	**1569 Kcal**	**1830 Kcal**	**2030 Kcal**	**2546 Kcal**	**3010 Kcal**

MEAL PLAN — THURSDAY

BREAKFAST	AVOCADO CHIA PROTEIN SHAKE *(page 62)*	1 SERVING
A.M. SNACK	NUTTY BLUEBERRY SNACK SQUARES *(page 150)*	1 SERVING
LUNCH	TACO TEMPEH SALAD *(page 77)*	1 SERVING
P.M. SNACK	CHOCOLATE. QUINOA AND ZUCCHINI MUFFINS *(page 127)*	1 SERVING
DINNER	TAHINI FALAFELS *(page 121)*	1 SERVING

CARBS	FAT	PROTEIN	CALORIES	SERVINGS	SERVINGS	SERVINGS	SERVINGS
16.6 g.	21.4 g.	30.1 g.	379 Kcal	1½	2	2	2
21.7 g.	13.1 g.	10.3 g.	246 Kcal	1	1	1	1
36.3 g.	23 g.	22.4 g.	441 Kcal	1	1	2	2
30.4 g.	19.4 g.	14.2 g.	354 Kcal	1	1	1	2
28 g.	7.3 g.	10.5 g.	220 Kcal	1	1	1	2
133 g.	**84.2 g.**	**87.5 g.**	**1640 Kcal**	**1829 Kcal**	**2019 Kcal**	**2459 Kcal**	**3033 Kcal**

MEAL PLAN — FRIDAY

BREAKFAST	OVERNIGHT COOKIE DOUGH OATS *(page 153)*	1 SERVING
A.M. SNACK	CRANBERRY PROTEIN SHAKE *(page 59)*	1 SERVING
LUNCH	LENTIL. LEMON AND MUSHROOM SALAD *(page 67)*	1 SERVING
P.M. SNACK	SAVORY SWEET LENTIL BITES *(page 151)*	1 SERVING
DINNER	SHAVED BRUSSEL SPROUT SALAD *(page 74)*	1 SERVING

CARBS	FAT	PROTEIN	CALORIES	SERVINGS	SERVINGS	SERVINGS	SERVINGS
22.7 g.	11.3 g.	30.7 g.	316 Kcal	1	1	1	1
19.9 g.	16.8 g.	23.6 g.	325 Kcal	1	1	1	1
28.1 g.	9.6 g.	15.8 g.	262 Kcal	2	2	2	3
30.6 g.	12.4 g.	7.4 g.	264 Kcal	1	1	2	3
45.3 g.	18.7 g.	11.5 g.	396 Kcal	1	1½	2	2
146.6 g.	**68.8 g.**	**89 g.**	**1563 Kcal**	**1825 Kcal**	**2023 Kcal**	**2485 Kcal**	**3011 Kcal**

Week 6: Meal Plan

Make sure to read the chapter 'Using the 14-day meal plan' before using this meal plan! *Shopping lists for each week of the complete 30-day meal plan can be found at: **https://tinyurl.com/grocerylists***

MEAL PLAN		MONDAY	
BREAKFAST	ALMOND EXPLOSION *(page 65)*		1 SERVING
A.M. SNACK	SPICY CHICKPEA POPPERS *(page 129)*		1 SERVING
LUNCH	RUBY RED ROOTBEET BURGER *(page 81)*		2 SERVINGS
P.M. SNACK	MATCHA ENERGY BALLS *(page 133)*		1 SERVING
DINNER	MUSHROOM PHO *(page 79)*		1 SERVING

CARBS	FAT	PROTEIN	CALORIES	SERVINGS	SERVINGS	SERVINGS	SERVINGS
29.5 g.	15 g.	25.4 g.	355 Kcal	1	1	2	2
21.5 g.	7.8 g.	9.1 g.	192 Kcal	2	3	3	4
46.4 g.	9.8 g.	11.2 g.	318 Kcal	2	2	3	2
21.3 g.	21.2 g.	14.6 g.	335 Kcal	1	1	1	2
57.3 g.	9.1 g.	17.8 g.	383 Kcal	1	1	1	1
176 g.	**62.9 g.**	**78.1 g.**	**1583 Kcal**	**1775 Kcal**	**1967 Kcal**	**2481 Kcal**	**3008 Kcal**

MEAL PLAN		TUESDAY					
BREAKFAST	POWERHOUSE PROTEIN SHAKE *(page 61)*				1 SERVING		
A.M. SNACK	CANDIED PROTEIN TRAIL MIX *(page 141)*				1 SERVING		
LUNCH	CREAMY SQUASH PIZZA *(page 84)*				1 SERVING		
P.M. SNACK	LENTIL RADISH SALAD *(page 71)*				1 SERVING		
DINNER	LASAGNA FUNGO *(page 85)*				1 SERVING		

CARBS	FAT	PROTEIN	CALORIES	SERVINGS	SERVINGS	SERVINGS	SERVINGS
30 g.	3.5 g.	26.3 g.	257 Kcal	1	1	2	3
19.5 g.	28 g.	14 g.	387 Kcal	1	1	1	1
62.5 g.	8.6 g.	18.4 g.	401 Kcal	1	1½	2	2
25.3 g.	10.7 g.	12.4 g.	247 Kcal	2	2	2	3
38 g.	9.2 g.	14.2 g.	292 Kcal	1	1	1	2
175.3 g.	**60 g.**	**85.3 g.**	**1584 Kcal**	**1831 Kcal**	**2031 Kcal**	**2488 Kcal**	**3027 Kcal**

MEAL PLAN		WEDNESDAY					
BREAKFAST	STRAWBERRY ORANGE SMOOTHIE *(page 60)*				1 SERVING		
A.M. SNACK	CRANBERRY VANILLA PROTEIN BARS *(page 145)*				1 SERVING		
LUNCH	COLORFUL PROTEIN POWER SALAD *(page 75)*				1 SERVING		
P.M. SNACK	GLUTEN-FREE ENERGY CRACKERS *(page 125)*				1 SERVING		
DINNER	SWEET POTATO QUESADILLAS *(page 93)*				1 SERVING		

CARBS	FAT	PROTEIN	CALORIES	SERVINGS	SERVINGS	SERVINGS	SERVINGS
29.3 g.	7.5 g.	25.6 g.	287 Kcal	1	1	1	2
22.9 g.	9.6 g.	16.1 g.	243 Kcal	2	2	2	2
64.8 g.	15.5 g.	22.3 g.	487 Kcal	1	1	2	2
10.3 g.	15.6 g.	6.9 g.	209 Kcal	1	2	2	3
54.8 g.	7.5 g.	10.6 g.	329 Kcal	1	1	1	1
182.1 g.	**55.7 g.**	**81.5 g.**	**1555 Kcal**	**1798 Kcal**	**2007 Kcal**	**2494 Kcal**	**2990 Kcal**

MEAL PLAN				THURSDAY			
BREAKFAST	TROPICAL PROTEIN SMOOTHIE *(page 58)*					1 SERVING	
A.M. SNACK	MOCHA CHOCOLATE BROWNIE BARS *(page 144)*					1 SERVING	
LUNCH	MANGO-TEMPEH WRAPS *(page 83)*					1 SERVING	
P.M. SNACK	NO-BAKE ALMOND-RICE TREATS *(page 142)*					2 SERVINGS	
DINNER	TACO TEMPEH SALAD *(page 77)*					1 SERVING	

CARBS	FAT	PROTEIN	CALORIES	SERVINGS	SERVINGS	SERVINGS	SERVINGS
44.4 g.	6.7 g.	27.9 g.	350 Kcal	1	1	1	2
17.3 g.	3.8 g.	27.3 g.	213 Kcal	1	1	1	2
31.3 g.	7.8 g.	15.7 g.	259 Kcal	1	1	1	1
26.4 g.	22.4 g.	18.6 g.	382 Kcal	3	4	4	4
36.3 g.	23 g.	22.4 g.	441 Kcal	1	1	2	2
155.7 g.	**63.7 g.**	**111.9 g.**	**1645 Kcal**	**1836 Kcal**	**2027 Kcal**	**2468 Kcal**	**3031 Kcal**

MEAL PLAN				FRIDAY			
BREAKFAST	HAZELNUT AND CHOCOLATE BARS *(page 149)*					1 SERVING	
A.M. SNACK	LEMON LIME PIE BARS *(page 134)*					1 SERVING	
LUNCH	HIGH PROTEIN BLACK BEAN DIP *(page 135)*					1 SERVING	
P.M. SNACK	SUNFLOWER PROTEIN BARS *(page 143)*					1 SERVING	
DINNER	STACKED N' SPICY PORTOBELLO BURGERS *(page 125)*					1 SERVING	

CARBS	FAT	PROTEIN	CALORIES	SERVINGS	SERVINGS	SERVINGS	SERVINGS
21.3 g.	14.2 g.	20.6 g.	296 Kcal	1	1	1	1
34.9 g.	10.7 g.	8.9 g.	272 Kcal	2	2	2	2
63 g.	6.6 g.	21.3 g.	398 Kcal	1	1	1	2
21.9 g.	6.8 g.	9.6 g.	188 Kcal	1	2	2	3
48.9 g.	16 g.	20.5 g.	421 Kcal	1	1	2	2
190 g.	**54.3 g.**	**80.9 g.**	**1575 Kcal**	**1874 Kcal**	**2035 Kcal**	**2456 Kcal**	**3042 Kcal**

Flavor Boosters

SPICES FOR TASTY RESULTS

When it comes to making your food taste better, spices are an absolute must. These ingredients are easy to find and store and can drastically change and improve the overall taste of meals, allowing you to get creative in the kitchen.

Spices can be added and changed according to personal taste and preference. By experimenting with flavors, you'll be able to create a wide variety of delicious, nutritional combinations with unique taste profiles. Spice up meals and staples to create a flavor profile that matches your or your family's interests.

Knowing and understanding how to use spices will allow you to be versatile in the kitchen. This goes for meals but also snack foods such as hummus, nut-based milk products, plant-based cheeses, chickpea poppers, and many other savory snacks.

Spice Ingredients

The spice recipes on the next pages include the following ingredients:

- Nutritional yeast
- Ground turmeric
- Ground cumin
- Ground coriander
- Curry powder
- Chili powder
- Mustard powder
- Cardamom powder
- Garam masala
- Vanilla extract
- Black pepper
- Cayenne pepper
- Paprika
- Ground cinnamon
- Ground cloves
- Nutmeg
- Ground ginger

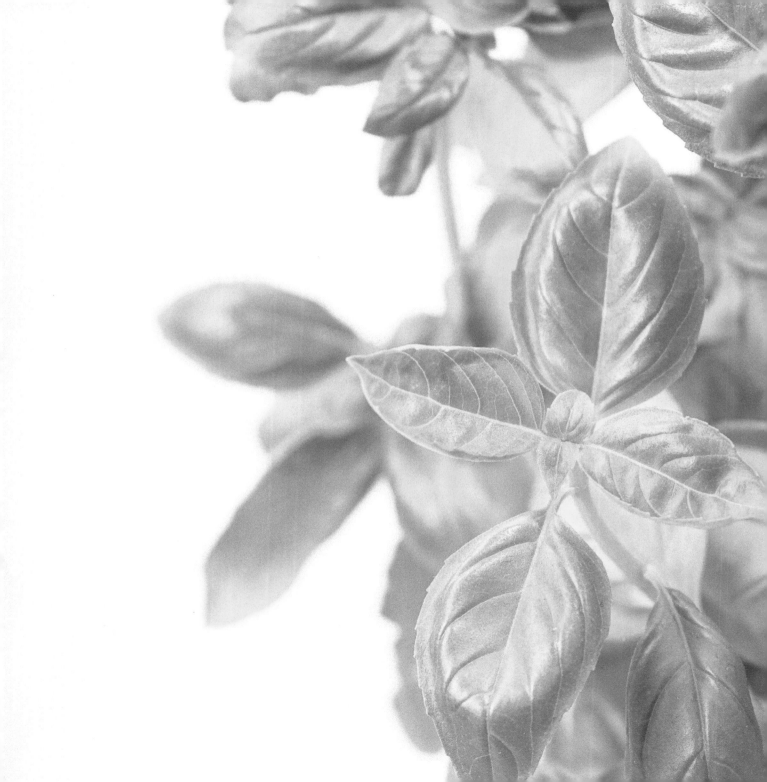

Berbere

This is an African spice blend made from:

- ½ cup chili powder or cayenne pepper
- ¼ cup sweet paprika
- 1 tbsp. salt
- ½ tsp. ground coriander
- 1 tsp. ground ginger
- ½ tsp. ground cardamom
- ½ tsp. ground fenugreek
- ¼ tsp. ground nutmeg
- ⅛ tsp. ground allspice
- ⅛ tsp. ground cloves.

Dukkah

An Egyptian spice made from a mix of:

- 1 cup toasted nuts
- ⅓ cup sesame seeds
- ⅔ cup hazelnuts
- 3 tbsp. coriander
- 3 tbsp. cumin
- 1 tsp. ground pepper

Harissa

A mixture of:

- 1 smoked red pepper
- ½ tsp. cumin
- ½ tsp. coriander
- ½ tsp. paprika
- 3 cloves garlic
- ½ tsp. sea salt
- ½ tsp. caraway
- 1 red onion

Ras el Hanout

A blend of:

- ¾ tsp. cumin
- ½ tsp. ginger
- ½ tsp. sea salt
- ½ tsp. black pepper
- 1¼ tsp. cinnamon
- ½ tsp. coriander
- ½ tsp. cayenne
- ¾ tsp. allspice

Chinese Five Spice

A mix of:

- 1 tsp. ground cinnamon
- 1 tsp. ground cloves
- ¼ tsp. fennel seed
- 1 tsp. star anise
- ¼ tsp. Szechuan peppercorns

Gomasio

A Japanese condiment that is a mix of:

- 2 cups toasted sesame seeds
- 1 tbsp. coarse salt

Togarashi

A mix of:

- 3 tbsp. chili pepper
- 3 tbsp. citrus peel
- 2 tbsp. sesame seeds
- 3 tbsp. Seaweed

Fines Herbes

A blend of fresh or dry herbs:

- 2 tbsp. chervil
- 2 tbsp. chives
- 4 tsps. tarragon
- 2 tbsp. parsley
- ½ tbsp. thyme
- 2 tbsp. chervil

Khmeli Suneli

A Georgian mix of:

- 2 tsps. fenugreek
- 1 tbsp. coriander
- 1 tbsp. savory
- ½ tsp. black peppercorns

Quatre Epices (Four spices)

A mix of:

- 2 tbsp. ground black and/or white pepper
- 1 tbsp. cloves
- 1 tbsp. nutmeg
- 1 tbsp. ginger

Curry Powder

A mix of:

- ¼ cup turmeric
- 2 tbsp. coriander
- 2 tbsp. cumin
- 2 tbsp. fenugreek
- ½ tsp. red pepper

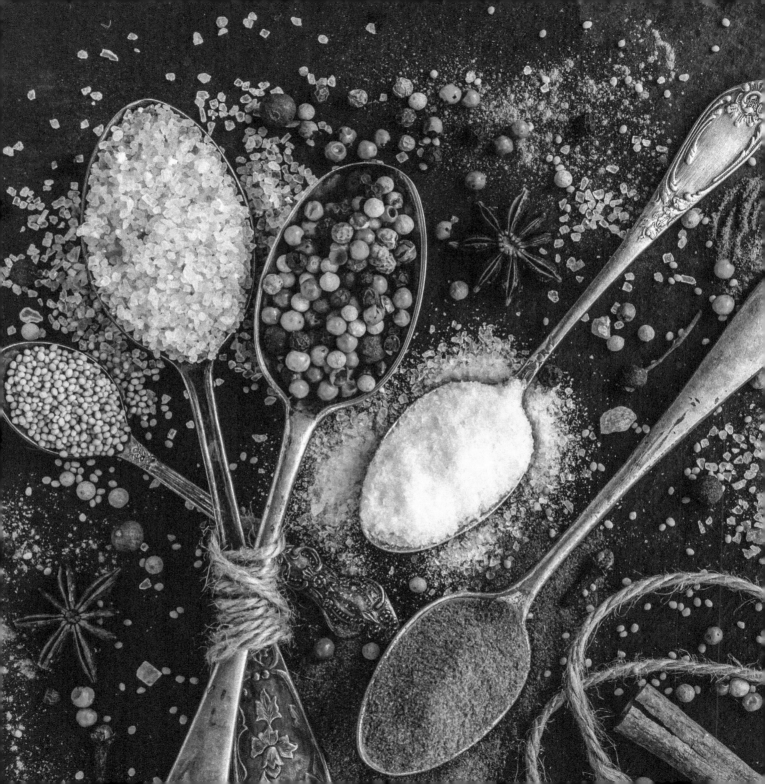

Garam Masala
A mix of:

- 2 tbsp. cinnamon
- 2 tbsp. cardamom
- 1 tbsp. cumin
- 2 tbsp. turmeric
- 1 tsp. mustard
- 1 tsp. fennel seed
- 2 red chilis

Panch Phoron
A mix of:

- 1 tbsp. fenugreek
- 1 tbsp. nigella
- 1 tbsp. cumin
- 1 tbsp. black mustard
- 1 tbsp. fennel seeds

Adobo
An all-purpose seasoning composed of:

- 1 tbsp. garlic
- 2 tbsp. oregano
- 3 tbsp. black pepper
- ¼ cup paprika
- 1 tbsp. garlic
- 2 tbsp. cumin

Chili Powder
A blend of:

- ancho chili
- 2 tbsp. paprika
- 1 ¼ tsps. cumin
- 2 tsps. Mexican oregano
- ¾ tsp. onion

Jerk Spice:
A spicy Jamaican composed of:

- 1 tsp. red and black pepper
- 1 tsp. allspice
- ¼ tsp. cinnamon
- 2 tsps. thyme
- 2 tsps. salt

Advieh
A mix of:

- 1 tsp. dried rose petals
- 1 tsp. cinnamon
- 1 tsp. cardamom
- 1 tsp. cloves
- 1 tsp. nutmeg
- ½ tsp. cumin

Baharat
A mixture of:

- 1 tsp. black pepper
- 2 tbsp. cumin
- ½ tsp. cinnamon
- ¼ tsp. cloves.
- ¼ tsp. cardamom
- 1 tsp. coriander

Za'atar
A mix of:

- 2 tbsp. thyme
- 1 tbsp. sesame seeds
- ¼ cup sumac
- 2 tbsp. oregano
- 2 tbsp. marjoram

Pickling Spice
A blend of:

- 2 tbsp. bay leaves
- 2 tbsp. mustard seeds
- 1 tsp. peppercorns
- 2 tsps. coriander
- 1 tbsp. allspice

Pumpkin Pie Spice
A mix of:

- 4 tbsp. cinnamon
- ½ tsp. nutmeg
- 2 tbsp. ginger
- 1 tsp. cloves

Mexican Spice
A blend of:

- 1 tbsp. cumin
- 1 tbsp. coriander
- 1 tbsp. paprika
- 1 tsp. oregano
- ½ tsp. chili
- ½ tsp. garlic powder

1. Easy Vegan BBQ Sauce

Serves: 1
2 | Prep Time: ~5 min |

Nutrition Information
(per serving)
- Calories: 12 kcal
- Carbs: 2.3 g.
- Fat: 0.1 g.
- Protein: 0.4 g.
- Fiber: 0.9 g.
- Sugar: 1.5 g.

INGREDIENTS:

- 1 8-oz. can sweet tomato sauce
- 2 tbsp. maple syrup
- 1 tbsp. apple cider vinegar
- 1½ tbsp. low-sodium soy sauce
- 1 tsp. chili flakes (or cayenne pepper)
- ½ tbsp. sweet paprika
- ½ tbsp. smoked paprika
- Optional: ½ tsp. dried oregano
- Optional: ½ tsp. liquid smoke

Total number of ingredients: 9

METHOD:

1. Take a medium-sized bowl and add all the ingredients, including the optional liquid smoke if desired.
2. Whisk the mixture until no lumps remain
3. Store for at least an hour in an airtight container or a sealable jar.
4. Enjoy!

STORAGE INFORMATION:

Storage	Temperature	Expiration date	Preparation
Airtight container M	Fridge at 38 – 40°F or 3°C	2 days after preparation	
Airtight container M	Freezer at -1°F or -20°C	60 days after preparation	Thaw at room temperature

Tip: Add less chili flakes or cayenne pepper if you're not a big fan of spicy flavors!

SAUCE RECIPES

2. Marinara Sauce

Nutrition Information
(per serving)
- Calories: 65 kcal
- Carbs: 4.9 g.
- Fat: 4.3 g.
- Protein: 1.5 g.
- Fiber: 1.3 g.
- Sugar: 3 g.

INGREDIENTS:
- 4 28-oz. cans diced tomatoes
- 1 cup fresh basil (chopped)
- 4 tbsp. olive oil
- 4 tbsp. nutritional yeast
- 6 medium garlic cloves (minced)
- 2 tsp. dried oregano
- 1½ tbsp. maple syrup
- ½ tsp. cayenne pepper
- Salt to taste

Total number of ingredients: 9

METHOD:
1. Heat a large pot over medium heat.
2. Add the olive oil and minced garlic; sauté for about 1 minute.
3. Continue by adding the diced tomatoes, maple syrup, cayenne pepper, and oregano. Taste and add salt accordingly.
4. Bring the mixture to a simmer. Reduce the heat to low and cover the pot. Simmer the ingredients for about 25 minutes.
5. Add the basil and nutritional yeast. Stir well. Add more water if necessary.
6. Add more spices or salt to taste.
7. Incorporate the sauce in a dish, or store for future use.

STORAGE INFORMATION:

Storage	Temperature	Expiration date	Preparation
Airtight container M	Fridge at 38 – 40°F or 3°C	2 days after preparation	
Airtight container M	Freezer at -1°F or -20°C	60 days after preparation	Thaw at room temperature

Tip: Add between 2 and 4 teaspoons of salt!

3. Enchilada Sauce

Nutrition Information
(per serving)
- Calories: 18 kcal
- Carbs: 0.6 g.
- Fat: 1.6 g.
- Protein: 0.1 g.
- Fiber: 0.2 g.
- Sugar: 0.1 g.

INGREDIENTS:
- 1½ tbsp. MCT oil
- ½ tbsp. chili powder
- ½ tbsp. whole wheat flour
- ½ tsp. ground cumin
- ¼ tsp. oregano (dried or fresh)
- ¼ tsp. salt (or to taste)
- 1 garlic clove (minced)
- 1 tbsp. tomato paste
- 1 cup vegetable broth (page 49)
- ½ tsp. apple vinegar
- ½ tsp. ground black pepper

Total number of ingredients: 11

METHOD:
1. Heat a small saucepan over medium heat.
2. Add the MCT oil and minced garlic to the pan and sauté for about 1 minute.
3. Mix the dry spices and flour in a medium bowl and pour the dry mixture into the saucepan.
4. Stir in the tomato paste immediately, and slowly pour in the vegetable broth, making sure that everything combines well.
5. When everything is mixed thoroughly, bring up the heat to medium-high until it gets to a simmer and cook for about 3 minutes or until the sauce becomes a bit thicker.
6. Remove the pan from the heat and add the vinegar with the black pepper, adding more salt and pepper to taste.

STORAGE INFORMATION:

Storage	Temperature	Expiration date	Preparation
Airtight container M	Fridge at 38 – 40°F or 3°C	2 days after preparation	
Airtight container M	Freezer at -1°F or -20°C	60 days after preparation	Thaw at room temperature

Tip: Add between 2 and 4 teaspoons of salt!

4. Mexican Salsa

METHOD:

1. Skin and seed tomatoes.
2. Halve the jalapeno; remove and discard stem, seeds, and placenta.
3. Cut the tomatoes and jalapeno into fine pieces and add to bowl.
4. Finely chop the cilantro and red onion and add to bowl.
5. Juice the lime into the bowl.
6. Mix the ingredients and season to taste with salt and black pepper.
7. Let sit for 1 hour before serving.

Nutrition Information
(per serving)

- Calories: 30 kcal.
- Carbs: 6.1 g.
- Fat: 0.3 g.
- Protein: 0.8 g.
- Fiber: 2.1 g.
- Sugar: 4 g.

NGREDIENTS:

- **4 large, firm tomatoes**
- **1 fresh jalapeno**
- **½ medium red onion**
- **2 tbsp. fresh cilantro (chopped)**
- **1 lime**
- **Salt & black pepper to taste**

Total number of ingredients: 6

STORAGE INFORMATION:

Storage	Temperature	Expiration date	Preparation
Airtight container M	Fridge at 38 – 40°F or 3°C	2 days after preparation	
Airtight container M	Freezer at -1°F or -20°C	60 days after preparation	Thaw at room temperature

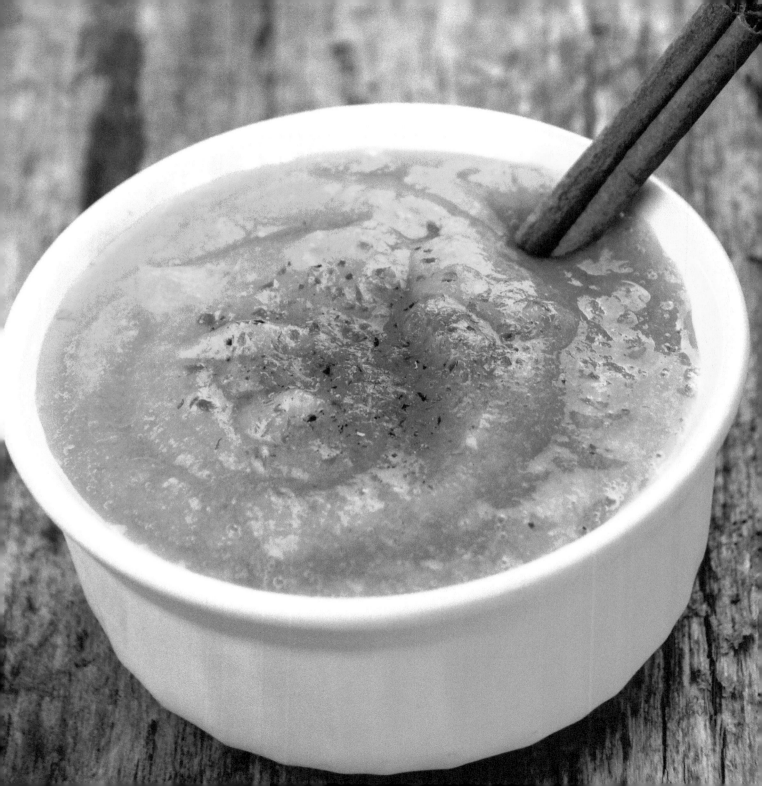

5. Apple Sauce

Nutrition Information
(per serving)
- Calories: 202 kcal.
- Carbs: 50.5 g.
- Fat: 0 g.
- Protein: 0 g.
- Fiber: 8.9 g.
- Sugar: 38 g.

INGREDIENTS:
- **4 Jazz apples (peeled, cored, and quartered)**
- **4 Red Delicious apples (peeled, cored, and quartered)**
- **½ cup water**
- **1 pinch salt**
- **Optional: ½ tsp. cinnamon**
- **Optional: 1 tbsp. lemon juice**

Total number of ingredients: 6

METHOD:

1. Put the apples into cold water for about 5 minutes.
2. Remove the apples from the water and further cut the quarters into slices.
3. Cook the slices of apple in a saucepan over medium heat with the water and salt.
4. Stir often and bring down to a simmer after it starts to cook.
5. After about 10 minutes of cooking, mash the apples while they are still simmering to create a sauce. Continue stirring and mashing further for about 20 minutes until you have a chunky apple sauce.
6. Add optional cinnamon and/or lemon juice if preferred.
7. Let it cool.
8. Blend if you prefer a smoother apple sauce.

STORAGE INFORMATION:

Storage	Temperature	Expiration date	Preparation
Airtight container M	Fridge at 38 – 40°F or 3°C	2 days after preparation	
Airtight container M	Freezer at -1°F or -20°C	60 days after preparation	Thaw at room temperature

6. Vegan Mayo

Nutrition Information
(per serving)
- Calories: 344 kcal.
- Carbs: 1.3 g.
- Fat: 37.5 g.
- Protein: 0 g.
- Fiber: 0.2 g.
- Sugar: 1.2 g.

INGREDIENTS:
- **1 cup MCT oil**
- **1 tsp. lemon juice**
- **½ cup almond milk**
- **1 tsp. agave nectar**
- **1 tsp. rice vinegar**
- **½ tsp. mustard (ground)**
- **Optional: 1 tsp. onion powder**
- **Optional: 1 tsp. chili powder**
- **Optional: 1 tsp. paprika powder**
- **Optional: 1 garlic clove**

Total number of ingredients: 10

METHOD:

1. Put the almond milk, agave nectar, rice vinegar, mustard, and if desired, the optional ingredients into a blender and blend.
2. Slowly add the MCT oil to the blender while blending to emulsify the oil and almond milk.
3. When the mixture starts to thicken, add the lemon juice.
4. Store in a sealable glass jar.

STORAGE INFORMATION:

Storage	Temperature	Expiration date	Preparation
Airtight container M	Fridge at 38 – 40°F or 3°C	4-5 days after preparation	
Airtight container M	Freezer at -1°F or -20°C	60 days after preparation	Thaw at room temperature

Thank you

Hopefully you've been able to find answers in this book and are well on your way to becoming a better plant-based athlete. Make follow the book's prescriptive diet and a better version of yourself will start to appear. If you have any questions regarding your nutrition protocol or workout plan, you can engage with a growing number of plant-based athletes in our exclusive Facebook group:

https://www.facebook.com/groups/PlantBasedAthletes

Also, if you enjoyed this book, we would like to ask you for a small favor. Would you be kind enough to leave an honest review of the book? Future readers and the team at HappyHealthyGreen would so appreciate it!

Did you discover any grammar mistakes, confusing explanations or inaccurate information? Send us an email! You can reach us at **info@happyhealthygreen.life**

We promise to get back at you as soon as time allows us. If this book requires a revision, we'll send you the updated eBook for free after the revised book is available.

CPSIA information can be obtained
at www.ICGtesting.com
Printed in the USA
BVHW022208250521
608082BV00006B/62

9 789492 788238